D0724326

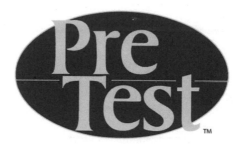

Medicine

PreTest™ Self-Assessment and Review

Notice

Medicine is an ever-changing science. As new research and clinical experience broaden our knowledge, changes in treatment and drug therapy are required. The authors and the publisher of this work have checked with sources believed to be reliable in their efforts to provide information that is complete and generally in accord with the standards accepted at the time of publication. However, in view of the possibility of human error or changes in medical sciences, neither the authors nor the publisher nor any other party who has been involved in the preparation or publication of this work warrants that the information contained herein is in every respect accurate or complete, and they disclaim all responsibility for any errors or omissions or for the results obtained from use of the information contained in this work. Readers are encouraged to confirm the information contained herein with other sources. For example and in particular, readers are advised to check the product information sheet included in the package of each drug they plan to administer to be certain that the information contained in this work is accurate and that changes have not been made in the recommended dose or in the contraindications for administration. This recommendation is of particular importance in connection with new or infrequently used drugs.

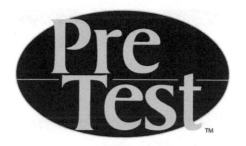

Medicine

PreTest™ Self-Assessment and Review
Eleventh Edition

Steven L. Berk, M.D.
Regional Dean
Professor of Medicine
Mirick-Myers Endowed Chair in Geriatric Medicine
Texas Tech University Health Science Center
School of Medicine at Amarillo

Marjorie R. Jenkins, M.D.
Associate Professor
Department of Internal Medicine
Department of Obstetrics and Gynecology
Texas Tech University Health Science Center
School of Medicine at Amarillo

William R. Davis, M.D.
Chairman and Associate Professor
Department of Internal Medicine
Texas Tech University Health Science Center
School of Medicine at Amarillo

Robert S. Urban, M.D.
Associate Professor
Department of Internal Medicine
Texas Tech University Health Science Center
School of Medicine at Amarillo

McGraw-Hill
Medical Publishing Division
New York   Chicago   San Francisco   Lisbon   London   Madrid   Mexico City
Milan   New Delhi   San Juan   Seoul   Singapore   Sydney   Toronto

The *McGraw·Hill* Companies

Medicine: PreTest™ Self-Assessment and Review, Eleventh Edition

1 2 3 4 5 6 7 8 9 0 DOC/DOC 0 9 8 7 6

ISBN 0-07-145553-1

This book was set in Berkeley by North Market Street Graphics.
The editor was Catherine A. Johnson.
The production supervisor was Sherri Souffrance.
Project management was provided by North Market Street Graphics.
The cover designer was Mary McKeon.
RR Donnelley was printer and binder.

This book is printed on acid-free paper.

Library of Congress Cataloging-in-Publication Data

Medicine : PreTest self-assessment and review.—11th ed. / [edited by] Steven L. Berk . . .
  [et al]
    p.; cm.
  Includes bibliographical references and index.
  ISBN 0-07-145553-1
    1. Medicine—Examinations, questions, etc. I. Berk, S.L. (Steven L.), 1949– .
  [DNLM: 1. Medicine—Examination Questions. W 18.2 M4914 2006]
  R834.5.B38 2006
  616.0076—dc22   2005058444

Contributors

Sina Aboutalebi, M.D.
Resident in Internal Medicine
Texas Tech University School of Medicine/Amarillo

Donald Loveman, M.D.
Professor and Regional Dean
Texas Tech University School of Medicine/Odessa

Stephen Kelleher, M.D.
Associate Professor of Internal Medicine
Texas Tech University School of Medicine/Amarillo

Student Reviewers

Anand Shah
University of Pennsylvania School of Medicine
Philadelphia, Pennsylvania
Class of 2007

Courtney Miller
Texas Tech University Health Science Center
School of Medicine
Amarillo, Texas
Class of 2006

Russ Womble
Texas Tech University Health Science Center
School of Medicine
Amarillo, Texas
Class of 2006

Contents

Introduction xi
Acknowledgments xiii

Infectious Disease

Questions I
Answers, Explanations, and References 17

Rheumatology

Questions 29
Answers, Explanations, and References 40

Pulmonary Disease

Questions 53
Answers, Explanations, and References 70

Cardiology

Questions 83
Answers, Explanations, and References 104

Endocrinology and Metabolic Disease

Questions 119
Answers, Explanations, and References 136

Gastroenterology

Questions 149
Answers, Explanations, and References 163

Nephrology

Questions 175
Answers, Explanations, and References 186

Hematology and Oncology

Questions. 195
Answers, Explanations, and References 211

Neurology

Questions. 227
Answers, Explanations, and References 240

Dermatology

Questions. 251
Answers, Explanations, and References 263

General Medicine and Prevention

Questions. 271
Answers, Explanations, and References 284

Allergy and Immunology

Questions. 295
Answers, Explanations, and References 300

Geriatrics

Questions. 305
Answers, Explanations, and References 311

Women's Health

Questions. 317
Answers, Explanations, and References 328

Bibliography 335
Index 337

Introduction

Medicine: PreTest™ Self-Assessment and Review, Eleventh Edition, is intended to provide medical students, as well as house officers and physicians, with a convenient tool for assessing and improving their knowledge of medicine. The 500 questions in this book are similar in format and complexity to those included in Step 2 of the United States Medical Licensing Examination (USMLE). They may also be a useful study tool for Step 3.

Each question in this book has a corresponding answer, a reference to a text that provides background for the answer, and a short discussion of various issues raised by the question and its answer. A listing of references for the entire book follows the last chapter.

To simulate the time constraints imposed by the qualifying examinations for which this book is intended as a practice guide, the student or physician should allot about one minute for each question. After answering all questions in a chapter, as much time as necessary should be spent reviewing the explanations for each question at the end of the chapter. Attention should be given to all explanations, even if the examinee answered the question correctly. Those seeking more information on a subject should refer to the reference materials listed or to other standard texts in medicine.

Acknowledgments

We would like to offer special thanks to:

Our spouses, Shirley Berk, Janet Davis, Joan Urban, and Stephen Jenkins for moral support and helpful suggestions

Our children, Jeremy Berk, Justin Berk, Abby Davis, Kyle Davis, David Urban, Elizabeth Urban, Catherine Urban, Katharine Jenkins, Matthew Jenkins, and Rebecca Jenkins

Texas Tech University School of Medicine at Amarillo—in the pursuit of excellence

Infectious Disease

Questions

DIRECTIONS: Each item below contains a question followed by suggested responses. Select the **one best** response to each question.

1. A 30-year-old male patient complains of fever and sore throat for several days. The patient presents to you today with additional complaints of hoarseness, difficulty breathing, and drooling. On examination, the patient is febrile and has inspiratory stridor. Which of the following is the best course of action?

a. Begin outpatient treatment with ampicillin
b. Culture throat for β-hemolytic streptococci
c. Admit to intensive care unit and obtain otolaryngology consultation
d. Schedule for chest x-ray
e. Obtain Epstein-Barr serology

2. A 70-year-old patient with long-standing type 2 diabetes mellitus presents with complaints of pain in the left ear with purulent drainage. On physical exam, the patient is afebrile. The pinna of the left ear is tender, and the external auditory canal is swollen and edematous. The peripheral white blood cell count is normal. Which of the following organisms is most likely to grow from the purulent drainage?

a. *Pseudomonas aeruginosa*
b. *Staphylococcus aureus*
c. *Candida albicans*
d. *Haemophilus influenzae*
e. *Moraxella catarrhalis*

3. A 25-year-old male student presents with the chief complaint of rash. There is no headache, fever, or myalgia. A slightly pruritic maculopapular rash is noted over the abdomen, trunk, palms of the hands, and soles of the feet. Inguinal, occipital, and cervical lymphadenopathy is also noted. Hypertrophic, flat, wartlike lesions are noted around the anal area. Laboratory studies show the following:

Hct: 40%
Hgb: 14 g/dL
WBC: 13,000/µL
Diff:
    Segmented neutrophils: 50%
    Lymphocytes: 50%

Which of the following is the most useful laboratory test in this patient?

a. Weil-Felix titer
b. Venereal Disease Research Laboratory (VDRL) test
c. Chlamydia titer
d. Blood cultures
e. Biopsy of lesions

4. A 20-year-old student has a macular rash, generalized lymphadenopathy, apthous ulcers, and gray-white plaques around the anal area. A dark-field examination demonstrates spirochetes. Which of the following is the treatment of choice for this patient?

a. Penicillin
b. Ceftriaxone
c. Tetracycline
d. Interferon α
e. Erythromycin

5. A 20-year-old female college student presents with a 5-day history of cough, low-grade fever (temperature 100°F), sore throat, and coryza. On exam, there is mild conjunctivitis and pharyngitis. Tympanic membranes are inflamed, and one bullous lesion is seen. Chest exam shows few basilar rales. Sputum Gram stain shows white blood cells without organisms. Laboratory findings are as follows:

Hct: 38
WBC: 12,000/μL
Lymphocytes: 50%
Mean corpuscular volume (MCV): 83 nL
Reticulocytes: 3% of red cells
CXR: bilateral patchy lower lobe infiltrates

Which of the following is the best method for confirmation of the diagnosis?

a. High titers of adenovirus
b. High titers of IgM cold agglutinins or complement fixation test
c. A positive silver methenamine stain
d. A positive blood culture for *Streptococcus pneumoniae*
e. Culture of sputum on chocolate media

6. The treatment of choice for a 20-year-old college student with a history of upper and lower respiratory symptoms, bullous myringitis, a negative sputum Gram stain, and patchy lower lobe infiltrates on chest x-ray is which of the following?

a. Erythromycin
b. Supportive therapy
c. Ceftriaxone
d. Cefuroxime
e. Penicillin

7. A 19-year-old male presents with a 1-week history of malaise and anorexia followed by fever and sore throat. On physical examination, the throat is inflamed without exudate. There are a few palatal petechiae. Cervical adenopathy is present. The liver is percussed at 12 cm and the spleen is palpable.

Throat culture: negative for group A streptococci
Hct: 38%
Hgb: 12 g/dL
Reticulocytes: 4%
WBC: 14,000/μL
    Segmented: 30%
    Lymphocytes: 60%
    Monocytes: 10%
Bilirubin total: 2.0 mg/dL (normal 0.2 to 1.2)
Lactic dehydrogenase (LDH) serum: 260 IU/L (normal 20 to 220)
Aspartate (AST): 40 U/L (normal 8 to 20 U/L)
Alanine (ALT): 35 U/L (normal 8 to 20 U/L)
Alkaline phosphatase: 40 IU/L (normal 35 to 125)

Which of the following is the most important initial test combination to order?

a. Liver biopsy and hepatitis antibody
b. Strep screen and ASO titer
c. Peripheral blood smear and heterophile antibody
d. Toxoplasmosis IgG and stool sample
e. Lymph node biopsy and cytomegalovirus serology

8. A 30-year-old male presents with right upper quadrant pain. He has been well except for an episode of diarrhea that occurred 4 months ago, just after he returned from a missionary trip to Mexico. He has lost 7 pounds. He is not having diarrhea. His blood pressure is 140/70, pulse 80, and temperature 99.5°F. On physical exam there is right upper quadrant tenderness without rebound. There is some radiation of the pain to the shoulder. The liver is percussed at 14 cm. There is no lower quadrant tenderness. Bowel sounds are normal and active. Which of the following is the most appropriate next step in evaluation of the patient?

a. Serology and ultrasound
b. Stool for ova and parasite
c. Blood cultures
d. Diagnostic aspirate
e. Empiric broad-spectrum antibiotic therapy

9. An 80-year-old male complains of a 3-day history of a painful rash extending over the left half of his forehead and down to his left eyelid. There are weeping vesicular lesions on physical examination. Which of the following is the most likely diagnosis?

a. Impetigo
b. Adult chickenpox
c. Herpes zoster
d. Coxsackie A virus
e. Herpes simplex

10. A 28-year-old female presents to her internist because of low-grade fever and acute lower abdominal pain. There is no nausea, vomiting, or diarrhea. On physical exam there is a temperature of 38.3°C and bilateral lower quadrant tenderness. There is no point tenderness or rebound. Bowel sounds are normal. Her white blood cell count is 15,000/μL and urinalysis shows no red or white blood cells. Serum β-hCG is not elevated. On pelvic examination an exudate is present and there is tenderness on motion of the cervix. Which of the following is the best next step in management?

a. Treatment with ceftriaxone and doxycycline
b. Endometrial biopsy
c. Surgical exploration
d. Dilation and curettage
e. Aztreonam

11. A 35-year-old male complains of inability to close his right eye. Examination shows facial nerve weakness of the upper and lower halves of the face. There are no other cranial nerve abnormalities and the rest of the neurological exam is normal. Examination of the heart, chest, abdomen, and skin show no additional abnormalities. There is no lymphadenopathy.

About one month previously the patient was seen by a dermatologist for a bull's-eye skin rash. The patient lives in Upstate New York and returned from a camping trip a few weeks before noting the rash. Which of the following is the most likely diagnosis?

a. Sarcoidosis
b. Idiopathic Bell's palsy
c. Lyme disease
d. Syphilis
e. Lacunar infarct

12. A 40-year-old airplane pilot is hospitalized with shortness of breath. He experienced fever, chills, and myalgias for several days prior to his breathing problems. He has returned from the Far East, where he visited Singapore and Hong Kong. He is found to be hypoxic, and chest x-ray shows diffuse opacification of both lung fields. Sputum and blood cultures are negative. Rapid testing for influenza A and B are also negative. Which of the following is the most important next step in management?

a. Begin treatment with amantadine
b. Respiratory isolation for coronavirus infection
c. Treatment for acute bacterial pneumonia
d. High resolution CT scan
e. Obtain ventilation-perfusion scan

13. A 25-year-old women is admitted with fever and hypotension. She has a 3-day history of feeling feverish. She has no history of chronic disease, but she uses tampons for heavy menses. She is acutely ill and on physical exam is found to have a diffuse erythematous rash extending to palms and soles. She is confused. Initial blood tests are as follows:

White blood cell count: 22,000/μL
Serum:
  Na++: 125 meq/L
  K+: 3.0 meq/L
  Ca++: 8.0 meq/ml
  Activated partial thromboplastin time: 65 (normal 21 to 36)
  Prothrombin time: 12 s
  Aspartate aminotransferase: 240 U/L
  Creatinine: 3.0 mg/dL
  Antinuclear antibodies: negative
  Anti-DNA antibodies: negative
  Serologic tests for RMSF, leptospirosis, measles: negative

   Which of the following best describes the pathophysiology of the disease process?

a. Acute bacteremia
b. Toxin-mediated inflammatory response syndrome
c. Exacerbation of connective tissue disease
d. Tick-borne rickettsial disease
e. Allergic reaction

14. You are a physician in charge of the patients who reside in a nursing home. Several of the patients have developed influenza-like symptoms, and the community is in the midst of an influenza A outbreak. None of the nursing home residents have received the influenza vaccine. Which course of action is most appropriate?

a. Give the influenza vaccine to all residents who do not have a contraindication to the vaccine (i.e., allergy to eggs)
b. Give the influenza vaccine to all residents who do not have a contraindication to the vaccine; also give amantadine for 2 weeks
c. Give amantadine alone to all residents
d. Do not give any prophylactic regimen

15. An elderly male develops fever 3 days after cholecystectomy. He becomes short of breath, and chest x-ray shows a new right lower lobe infiltrate. Sputum Gram stain shows gram-positive cocci in clumps, and preliminary culture results suggest staphylococci. Which of the following is the initial antibiotic of choice?

a. Penicillinase-resistant penicillin such as nafcillin
b. Linezolid
c. Antibiotic therapy should be based on the incidence of methicillin-resistant staphylococci in that hospital
d. Quinolones have become the drug of choice for pneumonia
e. Quinupristin-dalfopristin

16. A 30-year-old male with sickle cell anemia is admitted with cough, rusty sputum, and a single shaking chill. Physical examination reveals increased tactile fremitus and bronchial breath sounds in the left posterior chest. The patient is able to expectorate a purulent sample. Which of the following best describes the role of sputum Gram stain and culture?

a. Sputum Gram stain and culture lack the sensitivity and specificity to be of value in this setting
b. If the sample is a good one, sputum culture is useful in determining the antibiotic sensitivity pattern of the organism, particularly *Streptococcus pneumoniae*
c. Empirical use of antibiotics for pneumonia has made specific diagnosis unnecessary
d. There is no characteristic Gram stain in a patient with pneumococcal pneumonia

17. A recent outbreak of severe diarrhea is currently being investigated. Several adolescents developed bloody diarrhea, and one remains hospitalized with acute renal failure. A preliminary investigation has determined that all the affected ate at the same restaurant. The food they consumed was most likely to be which of the following?

a. Pork chops
b. Hamburger
c. Gefilte fish
d. Sushi
e. Soft-boiled eggs

18. A 40-year-old female nurse was admitted to the hospital because of fever to 103°F. Despite a thorough workup in the hospital for over 3 weeks, no etiology has been found, and she continues to have temperature spikes greater than 102°F. Which of the following statements about diagnosis is correct?

a. Chronic infection, malignancy, and collagen vascular disease are the most common explanations for this presentation
b. Influenza may also present in this manner
c. Lymphoma can be ruled out in the absence of palpable lymphadenopathy
d. SLE is an increasing cause for this syndrome
e. Factitious fever should be considered only in the patient with known psychopathology

19. You are counseling a 40-year-old male with newly diagnosed mitral valve insufficiency on the importance of receiving prophylactic antibiotics for certain procedures. Which of the following would not require such prophylaxis?

a. Cardiac catheterization
b. Prostatectomy
c. Cystoscopy
d. Tonsillectomy
e. Periodontal surgery

20. A previously healthy 25-year-old music teacher develops fever and a rash over her face and chest. The rash is itchy and on exam involves multiple papules and vesicles in varying stages of development. One week later she complains of cough and is found to have an infiltrate on x-ray. Which of the following is the most likely etiology of the infection?

a. *Streptococcus pneumoniae*
b. *Mycoplasma pneumoniae*
c. *Pneumocystis carinii*
d. Varicella virus
e. *Chlamydia psitacii*

21. A 22-year-old male complains of fever and shortness of breath. There is no pleuritic chest pain or rigors and no sputum production. A chest x-ray shows diffuse perihilar infiltrates. The patient worsens while on erythromycin. A silver methenamine stain shows cystlike structures. Which of the following is correct?

a. Definitive diagnosis can be made by serology
b. The organism will grow after 48 h
c. History will likely provide important clues to the diagnosis
d. Cavitary disease is likely to develop

22. A 22-year-old with the presumptive diagnosis of *Pneumocystis jiroveci* (formerly *carinii*) pneumonia is in no respiratory distress and is not hypoxic. Which of the following statements is correct?

a. Oral antibiotic therapy is never appropriate
b. Trimethoprim-sulfamethoxazole is the treatment of choice in the nonallergic patient
c. Concomitant corticosteroids should always be avoided
d. Tetracycline is more effective than erythromycin

23. A 25-year-old male from East Tennessee had been ill for 5 days with fever, chills, and headache when he noted a rash that developed on his palms and soles. In addition to macular lesions, petechiae are noted on the wrists and ankles. The patient has spent the summer camping. Which of the following is the most important fact to be determined in the history?

a. Exposure to contaminated springwater
b. Exposure to raw pork
c. Exposure to ticks
d. Exposure to prostitutes

24. A 19-year-old male has a history of athlete's foot but is otherwise healthy when he develops the sudden onset of fever and pain in the right foot and leg. On physical exam, the foot and leg are fiery red with a well-defined indurated margin that appears to be rapidly advancing. There is tender inguinal lymphadenopathy. The most likely organism to cause this infection is which of the following?

a. *Staphylococcus epidermidis*
b. *Tinea pedis*
c. *Streptococcus pyogenes*
d. Mixed anaerobic infection

25. An 18-year-old male has been seen in clinic for urethral discharge. He is treated with ceftriaxone, but the discharge has not resolved and the culture has returned as no growth. Which of the following is the most likely etiologic agent to cause this infection?

a. Ceftriaxone-resistant gonococci
b. *Chlamydia psittaci*
c. *Chlamydia trachomatis*
d. Herpes simplex

DIRECTIONS: Each group of questions below consists of lettered options followed by a set of numbered items. For each numbered item, select the **one** lettered option with which it is **most** closely associated. Each lettered option may be used once, more than once, or not at all.

Questions 26–29

Match the clinical description with the most likely organism.

a. *Streptococcus pneumoniae*
b. *Staphylococcus aureus*
c. Viridans streptococci
d. *Providencia stuartii*
e. *Actinomyces israelii*
f. *Haemophilus ducreyi*
g. *Neisseria meningitidis*
h. *Listeria monocytogenes*

26. A 30-year-old female with mitral valve prolapse and mitral regurgitant murmur develops fever, weight loss, and anorexia after undergoing a dental procedure.

27. An 80-year-old-male, hospitalized for hip fracture, has a Foley catheter in place when he develops shaking chills, fever, and hypotension.

28. A young man develops a painless, fluctuant purplish lesion over the mandible. A cutaneous fistula is noted after several weeks.

29. A sickle cell anemia patient presents with high fever, toxicity, signs of pneumonia, and stiff neck.

41. A recently diagnosed HIV-positive patient develops dyspnea, fever and sweats. Examination of the lungs is unremarkable.

42. A 40-year-old with advanced HIV disease and CD4 count of 75 cells/μL complains of blurred vision and floaters.

43. A 20-year-old homosexual male who has had headaches and change in personality presents with tonic-clonic seizure.

44. A nursing home patient with HIV disease develops fulminant diarrhea, rectal ulcerations, and shaking chills.

45. A 25-year-old female drug abuser presents for evaluation of a 20-day history of watery diarrhea. Pathogen is established by direct examination of stool.

Questions 46–50

For each of the patients with sexually transmitted diseases, select the treatment of choice.

a. Penicillin
b. Doxycycline
c. Ceftriaxone plus doxycycline
d. Metronidazole
e. Acyclovir
f. Aztreonam
g. Vancomycin
h. Meropenem

46. A 26-year-old sexually active male develops a urethral discharge for the second time in 1 year. Gram stain of the discharge shows many white blood cells and gram-negative kidney-bean-shaped diplococci.

47. A sexually active 25-year-old male develops a urethral discharge for the first time. Urethral smear shows white blood cells but no organisms, and culture is negative.

48. An 18-year-old sexually active male develops fever and malaise and notes painful blister-like lesions on the head of the penis.

49. A 30-year-old woman complains of vaginal discharge with vulvovaginal soreness and irritation. Wet preparation of discharge shows white blood cells and motile, flagellated pear-shaped organisms.

50. A sexually active male notes a single painless papule on the shaft of the penis. Its borders are raised and firm. Darkfield examination is positive.

Questions 51–54

Identify the antimicrobial agent associated with the adverse effects listed below.

a. Gentamicin *NM Block, ATN*
b. Imipenem *Seizure*
c. Tetracycline *Photosens*
d. Clindamycin
e. Azithromycin
f. Aztreonam
g. Trimethoprim

51. A vacationing 18-year-old woman develops a painful red rash after lying beside the swimming pool.

52. This 75-year-old male develops azotemia after treatment for a urinary tract infection. Urine examination shows renal tubular epithelial cells and muddy brown casts.

53. This 40-year-old male with myasthenia gravis is treated for gram-negative pneumonia. He suddenly develops weakness of respiratory musculature, flaccid paralysis, and dilated pupils.

54. A 55-year-old male is being treated for hospital-acquired pneumonia. He has a recent history of stroke. The patient develops a seizure on administration of the antibiotic.

Questions 55–60

Match the clinical description with the most likely etiologic agent.

a. *Candida albicans*
b. *Aspergillus flavus* – Fungus ball
c. *Coccidioides immitis*
d. Herpes simplex type 1
e. Herpes simplex type 2
f. Hantavirus
g. *Tropheryma whippelii*
h. Coxsackievirus B – URI → myocarditis
i. *Histoplasma capsulatum*
j. Human parvovirus
k. *Cryptococcus neoformans*

55. An HIV-positive patient develops fever and dysphagia; endoscopic biopsy shows yeast and hyphae.

56. A 50-year-old develops sudden onset of bizarre behavior. CSF shows 80 lymphocytes; magnetic resonance imaging shows temporal lobe abnormalities.

57. A patient with a previous history of tuberculosis now complains of hemoptysis. There is an upper lobe mass with a cavity and a crescent-shaped air-fluid level.

58. A Filipino patient develops a pulmonary nodule after travel through the American Southwest.

59. A 35-year-old male who had a fever, cough, and sore throat develops chest pain after several days, with diffuse ST segment elevations on ECG.

60. Overwhelming pneumonia with adult respiratory distress syndrome occurs on an Indian reservation in the Southwest following exposure to deer mice.

Infectious Disease

Answers

1. The answer is c. (*Kasper, pp 192–193.*) This patient, with the development of hoarseness, breathing difficulty, and stridor, is likely to have acute epiglottitis. Because of the possibility of impending airway obstruction, the patient should be admitted to an intensive care unit for close monitoring. The diagnosis can be confirmed by indirect laryngoscopy or soft tissue x-rays of the neck, which may show an enlarged epiglottis. Otolaryngology consult should be obtained. The most likely organism causing this infection is *Haemophilus influenzae*. Many of these organisms are β-lactamase-producing and would be resistant to ampicillin. The clinical findings are not consistent with the presentation of streptococcal pharyngitis. Lateral neck films would be more useful than a chest x-ray. Classic findings on lateral neck films would be the thumbprint sign.

2. The answer is a. (*Kasper, pp 188–189.*) Ear pain and drainage in an elderly diabetic patient must raise concern about malignant external otitis. The swelling and inflammation of the external auditory meatus strongly suggest this diagnosis. This infection usually occurs in older diabetics and is almost always caused by *P. aeruginosa*. *H. influenzae* and *M. catarrhalis* frequently cause otitis media, but not external otitis.

3. The answer is b. (*Kasper, pp 978–980.*) The diffuse rash involving palms and soles would in itself suggest the possibility of secondary syphilis. The hypertrophic, wartlike lesions around the anal area, called *condylomata lata,* are specific for secondary syphilis. The VDRL slide test will be positive in all patients with secondary syphilis. The Weil-Felix titer has been used as a screening test for rickettsial infection. In this patient, who has condylomata and no systemic symptoms, Rocky Mountain spotted fever would be unlikely. No chlamydial infection would present in this way. Blood cultures might be drawn to rule out bacterial infection such as chronic meningococcemia; however, the clinical picture is not consistent with a systemic bacterial infection.

4. The answer is a. (*Kasper, pp 978–980.*) Penicillin is the drug of choice for secondary syphilis. A positive darkfield examination in this patient confirms the diagnosis. Ceftriaxone and tetracycline are usually considered to be alternative therapies. Interferon α has been used in the treatment of condyloma acuminata, a lesion that can be mistaken for syphilitic condyloma.

5. The answer is b. (*Kasper, pp 1008–1009.*) This young woman presents with symptoms of both upper and lower respiratory infection. The combination of sore throat, bullous myringitis, and infiltrates on chest x-ray is consistent with infection due to *M. pneumoniae*. This minute organism is not seen on Gram stain. Neither *S. pneumoniae* nor *H. influenzae* would produce this combination of upper and lower respiratory tract symptoms. The patient is likely to have high titers of IgM cold agglutinins and a positive complement fixation test for mycoplasma. The low hematocrit and elevated reticulocyte count reflect a hemolytic anemia that can occur from mycoplasma infection. These IgM-class antibodies are directed to the I antigen on the erythrocyte membrane.

6. The answer is a. (*Kasper, pp 1009–1010*). The treatment of choice for mycoplasma infection is erythromycin. Newer macrolides such as azithromycin or clarithromycin are also effective. Treatment decreases the number of symptomatic days. Mycoplasma does not have a cell wall membrane, so neither penicillin nor ceftriaxone would be effective therapy.

7. The answer is c. (*Kasper, pp 1046–1047.*) This young man presents with classic signs and symptoms of infectious mononucleosis. In a young patient with fever, pharyngitis, lymphadenopathy, and lymphocytosis, the peripheral blood smear should be evaluated for atypical lymphocytes. A heterophile antibody test should be performed. The symptoms described in association with atypical lymphocytes and a positive heterophile test are virtually always due to Epstein-Barr virus. Neither liver biopsy nor lymph node biopsy is necessary. Workup for toxoplasmosis or cytomegalovirus infection or hepatitis B and C would be considered in heterophile-negative patients. Hepatitis does not occur in the setting of rheumatic fever, and an antistreptolysin O titer is not indicated.

8. The answer is a. (*Kasper, pp 1214–1217.*) The history and physical exam suggest amebic liver abscess. Symptoms usually occur 2 to 5 months after travel to an endemic area. Diarrhea often presents prior to the history of abdominal pain, but usually does not occur at the same time as the hepatic symptoms. The most common presentation for an amebic liver abscess is abdominal pain, usually RUQ. An indirect hemagglutination test is a sensitive assay and will be positive in 90 to 100% of patients. Ultrasound has a 75 to 85% sensitivity and shows abscess with well-defined margins. Stool will not show the trophozoite at this stage of the disease process. Blood cultures could be obtained to rule out pyogenic abscess, but the patient does not have signs of toxicity. Aspiration is usually not necessary unless rupture of abscess is imminent. Metronidazole remains the drug of choice for amebic liver abscess.

9. The answer is c. *(Kasper, pp 1042–1044.)* A painful vesicular rash that has a dermatomal distribution strongly suggests herpes zoster, although other viral pathogens may also cause vesicles. Herpes zoster may involve the eyelid when the first or second branch of the fifth cranial nerve is affected. Impetigo is a cellulitis caused by group A β-hemolytic streptococci. It often involves the face and can occur after an abrasion of the skin. Its distribution is not dermatomal, and while it may cause vesicles, they are usually small and are not weeping fluid. Chickenpox produces vesicles in various stages of development that are diffuse and produce more pruritus than pain. Coxsackievirus can produce a morbilliform vesiculopustular rash, often with a hemorrhagic component and with lesions of the throat, palms, and soles.

10. The answer is a. *(Kasper, pp 769–770.)* This patient presents with clinical criteria sufficient for the diagnosis of pelvic inflammatory disease, including lower quadrant tenderness, cervical motion tenderness, and adnexal tenderness. Fever and mucopurulent discharge are additional evidence for the diagnosis. Treatment requires antibiotic therapy. Ceftriaxone and doxycycline are one recommended regimen that would cover both *N. gonorrheae* and *C. trachomatis*. Endometrial biopsy can provide definitive diagnosis, but it is unnecessary except when patients do not respond to therapy or have atypical presentations. At times, surgical emergencies may mimic the disease and even require hospitalization for further observation. The specific findings of cervical motion tenderness, discharge, and bilateral tenderness all distinguish PID from appendicitis in this patient.

11. The answer is c. *(Kasper, pp 995–998, 109–110.)* Symptoms and time course are consistent with stage 2 Lyme disease. A few weeks after a camping trip and presumptive exposure to the *Ixodes* tick, the patient developed a rash that is described to be consistent with erythema chronicum migrans. Secondary neurologic, cardiac, or arthritic symptoms occur weeks to months after the rash. A facial nerve palsy is one of the more common signs of stage 2 Lyme disease. Sarcoidosis is in the differential of facial palsy, but there are no other signs or symptoms to suggest this disease. Syphilis always needs to be considered in the same differential with Lyme disease, but the rash described would be atypical, and there are no other neurologic findings of syphilis. Lacunar infarct would not cause the lower motor neuron findings.

12. The answer is b. *(Kasper, pp 1060–1062.)* Severe acute respiratory syndrome (SARS) was first recognized in Mainland China in 2002. It eventually spread to 26 countries on five continents and affected 8000 patients. The initial symptoms of the disease are similar to influenza, with myalgias, fever, chills, and malaise. The disease progresses to shortness of breath and ARDS, and many patients require mechanical ventilation. The organism is now known to be a coronavirus (SARS-CoV). Treatment is supportive with no antiviral therapy yet proven. Respiratory isolation is extremely important, as the disease spreads through hospitals, affecting health care workers and other hospital employees. Chest x-rays in the advanced disease show a diffuse opacification of the lungs. High-resolution CT may demonstrate abnormalities prior to them being seen on standard x-ray but would not be helpful in this case. Bacterial superinfection should be ruled out, but cultures of blood and sputum are negative.

13. The answer is b. *(Kasper, pp 112, 304–305, 819.)* The disease process described is most consistent with toxic shock syndrome, an inflammatory response syndrome characterized by hypotension, fever, and multiorgan involvement. It can occur in healthy women who use tampons. TSST-1 is a toxin produced by *S. aureus* that is responsible for activating superantigens such as tumor necrosis factor and interleukin-1. Symptoms include confusion, as has occurred in this patient, in addition to diarrhea, myalgias, nausea and vomiting, and syncope. In addition to fever and hypotension there is a diffuse rash initially appearing on the trunk but spreading to palms of the hand and soles of the feet. Desquamation occurs a week after initial appearance of the rash. There are many potential laboratory abnormalities as manifestations of multiorgan involvement. These include azotemia, coagulopathy with abnormal aPTT, and electrolyte abnormalities, including hyponatremia, hypocalcemia, and hypokalemia. Liver function tests show hyperbilirubunemia and elevated alanine aminotransferase.

The disease is not a bacteremia, although it is precipitated by localized staphylococcal or sometimes streptococcal infection. Toxic shock syndrome sometimes mimics diseases that cause multiorgan involvement, such as systemic lupus or Rocky Mountain spotted fever. Serological studies for these diseases were negative in this patient.

14. The answer is b. *(Kasper, p 1070.)* Influenza A is a potentially lethal disease in the elderly and chronically debilitated patient. In institutional settings such as nursing homes, outbreaks are likely to be particularly severe. Thus, prophylaxis is extremely important in this setting. All residents should receive the vaccine unless they have known egg allergy (patients can choose to decline the vaccine). Since protective antibodies to the vaccine will not develop for 2 weeks, amantadine can be used for protection against influenza A during the interim 2-week period. A reduced dose is given to elderly patients. Rimantidine and oseltamivir are also used in prophylaxis.

15. The answer is c. *(Kasper, p 1541.)* In the treatment of hospital-acquired staphylococcal pneumonia, the incidence of methicillin-resistant staph (MRSA) in the local facility will be very important. In most hospitals, methicillin-resistant staph is common enough to require initial therapy with vancomycin. Oxacillin would be the drug of choice only if the incidence of methicillin-resistant staph is very low. Quinolones are often useful in the treatment of community-acquired pneumonia, but they would not be effective against methicillin-resistant staph. Linezolide is used when there is a contraindication to vancomycin.

16. The answer is b. *(Kasper, pp 1530–1533.)* The Infectious Disease Society of America's guidelines on the treatment of community-acquired pneumonia still recommend the use of sputum Gram stain and culture. This is particularly important in the era of multi-antibiotic-resistant *S. pneumoniae*. Sputum culture and sensitivity can direct specific antibiotic therapy for the patient as well as provide epidemiologic information for the community as a whole. A good sputum sample showing many polymorphonuclear leuko-cytes and few squamous epithelial cells can give important clues to etiology. A Gram stain that shows gram-positive lancet-shaped diplococci intracellularly is good evidence for pneumococcal infection. Empirical antibiotic therapy becomes more difficult in community-acquired pneumonia as more pathogens are recognized and as the pneumococcus develops resistance to penicillin, macrolides, and even quinolones.

17. The answer is b. *(Kasper, p 878.)* The outbreak described is similar to those caused by *Escherichia coli* O157:H7. Ingestion of and infection with this organism may result in a spectrum of illnesses, including mild diarrhea, hemorrhagic colitis with bloody diarrhea, acute renal failure, and hemolytic uremic syndrome. Infection has been associated with ingestion of contaminated beef (in particular ground beef), ingestion of raw milk, and contamination via the fecal-oral route. Cooking ground beef until it is no longer pink is an effective means of preventing infection, as are hand washing and pasteurization of milk.

18. The answer is a. *(Kasper, pp 116–118.)* Patients may develop fever as a result of infectious or noninfectious diseases. The term *fever of unknown origin* (FUO) is applied when significant fever persists without a known cause after an adequate evaluation. Several studies have found the leading causes of FUO to include infections, malignancies, collagen vascular diseases, and granulomatous diseases. As the ability to more rapidly diagnose some of these diseases increases, their likelihood of causing undiagnosed persistent fever lessens. Infections such as intraabdominal abscesses, tuberculosis, hepatobiliary disease, endocarditis (especially if the patient had previously taken antibiotics), and osteomyelitis may cause FUO. In immunocompromised patients, such as those infected with HIV, a number of opportunistic infections or lymphomas may cause fever and escape early diagnosis. Self-limited infections such as influenza should not cause fever that persists for many weeks. Neoplastic diseases such as lymphomas and some solid tumors (e.g., hypernephroma and primary or metastatic disease of the liver) are associated with FUO. A number of collagen vascular diseases may cause FUO. Since conditions such as systemic lupus erythematosus are more easily diagnosed today, they are less frequent causes of this syndrome. Adult Still's disease, however, is often difficult to diagnose. Other causes of FUO include granulomatous diseases (i.e., giant cell arteritis, regional enteritis, sarcoidosis, and granulomatous hepatitis), drug fever, and peripheral pulmonary emboli. Factitious fever is most common among young adults employed in health-related positions. A prior psychiatric history or multiple hospitalizations at other institutions may be clues to this condition. Such patients may induce infections by self-injection of non-sterile material, with resultant multiple abscesses or polymicrobial infections. Alternatively, some patients may manipulate their thermometers. In these cases, a discrepancy between temperature and pulse or between oral temperature and witnessed rectal temperature will be observed.

19. The answer is a. *(Kasper, pp 739, 804.)* Although no evidence exists that prophylactic antibiotic therapy prevents endocarditis, prophylaxis is recommended for all procedures that may generate bacteremias. Following cardiac catheterization, blood cultures obtained from a distal vein are rarely positive. Thus, prophylactic antibiotics are not currently recommended for cardiac catheterization. Bacteremia commonly occurs following other procedures such as periodontal surgery, tonsillectomy, and prostate surgery.

20. The answer is d. *(Kasper, pp 1042–1043.)* Varicella pneumonia develops in about 20% of adults with chickenpox. It occurs 3 to 7 days after the onset of the rash. The hallmark of the chickenpox rash is papules, vesicles, and scabs in various stages of development. Fever, malaise, and itching are usually part of the clinical picture. The differential can include some coxsackievirus and echovirus infections, which might present with pneumonia and vesicular rash. Rickettsialpox, a rickettsial infection, has also been mistaken for chickenpox.

21. The answer is c. *(Kasper, pp 1194–1195.)* Patients with *Pneumocystis jiroveci* (formerly *carinii*) frequently present with shortness of breath and no sputum production. The interstitial pattern of infiltrates on chest x-ray distinguishes the pneumonia from most bacterial infections. Diagnosis is made by review of silver methenamine stain. Serology is not sensitive or specific enough for routine use. The organism does not grow on any media. Cavitation can occur but is quite unusual. The history is likely to suggest a risk factor for HIV disease.

22. The answer is b. *(Kasper, pp 1195–1196.)* Trimethoprim-sulfa is the drug of choice for *P. jiroveci* pneumonia in the nonallergic patient. Oral therapy is recommended for mild to moderate disease. Prednisone has been shown to improve the mortality rate in moderate to severe disease when the P_{O_2} is less than 70 mmHg. Neither tetracycline nor erythromycin has any effect on the organism.

23. The answer is c. (*Kasper, pp 108–109, 999–1000.*) The rash of Rocky Mountain spotted fever (RMSF) occurs about 5 days into an illness characterized by fever, malaise, and headache. The rash may be macular or petechial, but almost always spreads from the ankles and wrists to the trunk. The disease is most common in spring and summer. North Carolina and East Tennessee have a relatively high index of disease. RMSF is a rickettsial disease with the tick as the vector. About 80% of patients will give a history of tick exposure. Doxycycline is considered the drug of choice, but chloramphenicol is preferred in pregnancy because of the effects of tetracycline on fetal bones and teeth. Overall mortality from the infection is now about 5%.

24. The answer is c. (*Kasper, pp 824–825, 827.*) Erysipelas, the cellulitis described, is typical of infection caused by *S. pyogenes* group A β-hemolytic streptococci. There is often a preceding event such as a cut in the skin, dermatitis, or superficial fungal infection that precedes this rapidly spreading cellulitis. Anaerobic cellulitis is more often associated with underlying diabetes. *S. epidermidis* does not cause rapidly progressive cellulitis. *Staphylococcus aureus* can cause cellulitis that is difficult to distinguish from erysipelas, but it is usually more focal and likely to produce furuncles, or abscesses.

25. The answer is c. (*Kasper, pp 1011–1012.*) About half of all cases of nongonococcal urethritis are caused by *C. trachomatis*. *Ureaplasma urealyticum* and *Trichomonas vaginalis* are rarer causes of urethritis. Herpes simplex would present with vesicular lesions and pain. *C. psittaci* is the etiologic agent in psittacosis. All gonococci are susceptible to ceftriaxone at recommended doses.

26–29. The answers are 26-c, 27-d, 28-e, 29-a. (*Kasper, pp 197, 732, 810, 885, 937.*) The 30-year-old-female with mitral valve prolapse has developed subacute bacterial endocarditis. The likely etiologic agent is a viridans streptococci. Viridans streptococci cause most cases of subacute bacterial endocarditis. No other agent listed is likely to cause this infection. The 80-year-old-male with a Foley catheter in place has developed a nosocomial infection likely secondary to urosepsis. *Providencia* species frequently cause urinary tract infection in the hospitalized patient. The young man with a fluctuant lesion and fistula over the mandible presents a classic picture of cervicofacial actinomycosis. The sickle cell anemia patient who presents with concomitant pneumonia and meningitis has overwhelming infection with *S. pneumoniae* due to functional asplenia. *S. pneumoniae* causes a particularly severe infection associated with sickle cell disease.

30–33. The answers are 30-f, 31-a, 32-c, 33-e. *(Kasper, pp 1051, 1058, 1063, 1069.)* Amantadine has been shown to alter the course of influenza A favorably, particularly when begun within 48 h of the start of symptoms. The HIV-positive patient with a low CD4 count and visual blurring has developed cytomegalovirus retinitis. Ganciclovir is the drug of choice (foscarnet has also been used effectively). Interferon α has been approved for intralesional therapy of condyloma acuminatum (venereal warts caused by papillomavirus). Ribavirin improves mortality in mechanically ventilated infants with RSV infection.

34–36. The answers are 34-b, 35-g, 36-f. *(Kasper, pp 1182–1183, 1188–1189, 1190.)* Blastomycosis presents with signs and symptoms of chronic respiratory infection. The organism has a tendency to produce skin lesions in exposed areas that become crusted, ulcerated, or verrucous. Bone pain is caused by osteolytic lesions. Mucormycosis is a zygomycosis that originates in the nose and paranasal sinuses. Sinus tenderness, bloody nasal discharge, and obtundation occur usually in the setting of diabetic ketoacidosis. *Aspergillus* can result in several different infectious processes, including aspergilloma, disseminated *Aspergillus* in the immunocompromised patient, or allergic bronchopulmonary aspergillosis. Bronchopulmonary aspergillosis is the most likely diagnosis in the young woman with asthma and eosinophilia. Bronchial plugs, often filled with hyphal forms, result in repeated infiltrates and exacerbation of wheezing.

37–40. The answers are 37-c, 38-d, 39-e, 40-b. *(Kasper, pp 109, 304–305, 816–817, 819, 853–853, 1046, 1055–1056.)* Parvovirus B19 is the agent responsible for erythema infectiosum, also known as fifth disease. This disease most commonly affects children between the ages of 5 and 14 years, but it can also occur in adults. The disease is characterized by a slapped-cheek rash, which may follow a prodrome of low-grade fever. A diffuse lacelike rash may also occur. Complications in adults include arthralgias, arthritis, aplastic crisis in patients with chronic hemolytic anemia, spontaneous abortion, and hydrops fetalis. Desquamation of the skin usually occurs during or after recovery from toxic shock syndrome (associated with a toxin produced by *S. aureus*). Peeling of the skin is also seen in Kawasaki disease, scarlet fever, and some severe drug reactions. Petechial rashes are often seen with potentially life-threatening infections, including meningococcemia, gonococcemia, rickettsial disease, infective endocarditis, atypical measles, and disseminated intravascular coagulation (DIC) associated with sepsis. Infectious mononucleosis is the usual manifestation of infection with Epstein-Barr virus. Since it is a viral disease, antibiotic therapy is not indicated. A diffuse maculopapular rash has been observed in over 90% of patients with infectious mononucleosis who are given ampicillin. The rash does not represent an allergic reaction to β-lactam antibiotics.

41–45. The answers are 41-a, 42-d, 43-b, 44-e, 45-c. *(Kasper, pp 1104–1107, 1109–1110, 1117–1119.)* Pneumonia due to *P. carinii* was among the first recognized manifestations of AIDS. The disease presents insidiously with dyspnea on exertion and nonproductive cough. The chest radiograph typically shows a diffuse bilateral interstitial pattern, but physical exam is often normal. Cytomegalovirus (CMV) occurs later in the course of AIDS, when the CD4 count is below 100 white cells per μL. Blurring of vision is the first sign of retinitis, which may lead to blindness if untreated. CMV may also cause pneumonitis, adrenalitis, and hepatitis, as well as colitis with significant diarrhea. The protozoan *Cryptosporidium* may cause a prolonged diarrhea that leads to malabsorption and wasting. Diarrhea may be the initial manifestation of HIV disease, and *Cryptosporidium* is the most likely etiology. The intracellular protozoan can be diagnosed by direct examination of the stool, with special concentration or staining techniques or both. *Salmonella* infections have been recognized with increased frequency in patients with HIV. These patients are prone to more severe disease such as fulminant diarrhea or may have bacteremia without GI symptoms. Headaches, personality changes, ataxia, and focal neurologic findings require evaluation for brain abscess, particularly secondary to *Toxoplasma gondii*. Seizures may be the first manifestation of tox-oplasmosis and may be the first manifestation of HIV disease.

46–50. The answers are 46-c, 47-b, 48-e, 49-d, 50-a. *(Kasper, pp 860–861, 983–985, 1040–1041, 1252.)* Treatment of gonococcal infections should be guided by the increasing frequency of antibiotic-resistant *Neisseria gonorrhoeae* and high frequency of co-infection with *Chlamydia trachomatis*. Because of the increased frequency of resistance to penicillin and tetracyclines, ceftriaxone is recommended as the treatment of choice. Doxycycline is added to treat chlamydial and other causes of nongonococcal urethritis. In cases in which gonorrhea has been ruled out, doxycycline or azithromycin may be used for the treatment of urethritis. First episodes of genital herpes may be particularly severe. Oral acyclovir will accelerate the healing but will not reduce the risk of recurrence once the drug is stopped. Trichomoniasis is usually diagnosed by a wet preparation microscopic examination or by culture. Both the patient and sexual partner should be treated with metronidazole. Penicillin remains the drug of choice for treatment of syphilis. The route of administration and duration of therapy depend on the stage of disease and presence of CNS involvement and may also be influenced by the HIV serostatus of the patient.

51–54. The answers are 51-c, 52-a, 53-a, 54-b. *(Kasper, pp 801–802.)* The tetracyclines are associated with photosensitization, and patients taking these antibiotics should be warned about exposure to the sun. Imipenem, a carbapenem, may cause central nervous system toxicity such as seizures, especially when administered at high dosages. Patients with previous CNS pathology are most at risk. The major toxicity of gentamicin, an aminoglycoside, is acute tubular necrosis; thus, drug levels should be closely monitored. This class of drugs can also produce neuromuscular blockade, especially when administered with concomitant neuromuscular blocking agents or to patients with impairment of neuromuscular transmission, such as myasthenia gravis.

55–60. The answers are 55-a, 56-d, 57-b, 58-c, 59-h, 60-f. *(Kasper, pp 1038, 1055–1056, 1144–1146, 1172, 1180–1181, 1186–1187, 1188, 1413, 2480–2483.)* There are several causes for dysphagia in the HIV-positive patient, including *C. albicans*, herpes simplex, and cytomegalovirus. The

69. A 22-year-old male develops the insidious onset of low back pain improved with exercise and worsened by rest. There is no history of diarrhea, conjunctivitis, urethritis, rash, or nail changes. On exam the patient has loss of mobility with respect to lumbar flexion and extension. He has a kyphotic posture. A plain film of the spine shows widening and sclerosis of the sacroiliac joints. Some calcification is noted in the anterior spinal ligament. Which of the following best characterizes this patient's disease process?

a. He is most likely to have acute lumbosacral back strain and requires bed rest
b. The patient has a spondyloarthropathy, most likely ankylosing spondylitis
c. The patient is likely to die from pulmonary fibrosis and extrathoracic restrictive lung disease
d. A rheumatoid factor is likely to be positive
e. A colonoscopy is likely to show Crohn's disease

70. A 20-year-old woman has developed low-grade fever, a malar rash, and arthralgias of the hands over several months. High titers of anti-DNA antibodies are noted, and complement levels are low. The patient's white blood cell count is 3000/μL, and platelet count is 90,000/μL. The patient is on no medications and has no signs of active infection. Which of the following statements is correct?

a. If glomerulonephritis, severe thrombocytopenia, or hemolytic anemia develops, high-dose glucocorticoid therapy would be indicated
b. Central nervous system symptoms will occur within 10 years
c. The patient can be expected to develop Raynaud's phenomenon when exposed to cold
d. The patient will have a false-positive test for syphilis
e. The disease process described is an absolute contraindication to pregnancy

71. A 45-year-old woman has pain in her fingers on exposure to cold, arthralgias, and difficulty swallowing solid food. Of the following tests, which, if positive, would be most supportive of a definitive diagnosis?

a. Rheumatoid factor
b. Antinucleolar antibody
c. ECG
d. BUN and creatinine
e. Reproduction of symptoms and findings by immersion of hands in cold water

72. A 20-year-old male complains of arthritis and eye irritation. He has a history of burning on urination. On exam, there is a joint effusion of the right knee and a dermatitis of the glans penis. Which of the following is correct?

a. *Neisseria gonorrhoeae* is likely to be cultured from the glans penis
b. The patient is likely to be rheumatoid factor–positive
c. An infectious process of the GI tract may precipitate this disease
d. An ANA is very likely to be positive

73. A 43-year-old man with diabetes and cardiomegaly has had an attack of pseudogout. He should be evaluated for which of the following?

a. Renal disease
b. Hemochromatosis
c. Peptic ulcer disease
d. Lyme disease
e. Inflammatory bowel disease

74. A 75-year-old male complains of headache. On one occasion he transiently lost vision in his right eye. He also complains of aching in the shoulders and neck. There are no focal neurologic findings. Carotid pulses are normal without bruits. Laboratory data show a mild anemia. Erythrocyte sedimation rate is 85. Which of the following is the best approach to management?

a. Begin glucocorticoid therapy and arrange for temporal artery biopsy
b. Schedule biopsy and begin corticosteroids based on biopsy results and clinical course
c. Schedule carotid angiography
d. Follow ESR and consider further studies if it remains elevated
e. Start aspirin and defer any invasive studies unless further symptoms develop

75. A 55-year-old man with psoriasis has been troubled by long-standing destructive arthritis involving the hands, wrists, shoulders, knees, and ankles. Hand films demonstrate pencil-in-cup deformities. He has been treated with naproxen 1 gm BID, sulfasalazine 1 g bid, prednisone 5 mg qd, and methotrexate 17.5 mg once a week without substantive improvement. Which of the following treatments is most likely to provide long-term benefit?

a. Cyclophosphamide
b. Addition of folic acid supplementation
c. Oral cyclosporine
d. Tumor necrosis factor inhibitor
e. Higher-dose steroids in the range of 20 mg of prednisone per day

76. A 65-year-old male develops the onset of severe knee pain over 24 hours. The knee is red, swollen, and tender. He has a history of diabetes mellitus and cardiomyopathy. An x-ray of the knee shows linear calcification. Definitive diagnosis is best made by which of the following?

a. Serum uric acid
b. Serum calcium
c. Arthrocentesis and identification of positively birefringent rhomboid crystals
d. Rheumatoid factor

77. A 35-year-old woman complains of aching all over. She says she sleeps poorly and all her muscles and joints hurt. Symptoms have progressed over several years. She reports she is desperate because pain and weakness often cause her to drop things. Physical exam shows multiple points of tenderness over the neck, shoulders, elbows, and wrists. There is no joint swelling or deformity. A complete blood count and erythrocyte sedimentation rate are normal. Rheumatoid factor is negative. Which of the following is the best therapeutic option in this patient?

a. Amitriptyline at bedtime
b. Prednisone
c. Weekly methotrexate
d. Hydroxycholoquine
e. Stretching exercises

78. A 70-year-old female with mild dementia complains of unilateral groin pain. There is some limitation of motion in the right hip. Which of the following is the most appropriate first step in evaluation?

a. CBC and erythrocyte sedimentation rate
b. Rheumatoid factor
c. X-ray of right hip
d. Bone scan

79. A 65-year-old woman who has a 12-year history of symmetrical polyarthritis is admitted to the hospital. Physical examination reveals splenomegaly, ulcerations over the lateral malleoli, and synovitis of the wrists, shoulders, and knees. There is no hepatomegaly. Laboratory values demonstrate a white blood cell count of 2500/μL and a rheumatoid factor titer of 1:4096. This patient's white blood cell differential count is likely to reveal which of the following?

a. Pancytopenia
b. Lymphopenia
c. Granulocytopenia
d. Lymphocytosis
e. Basophilia

80. A 42-year-old woman presents with a 4-month history of fatigue and arthralgias. She complains of 2-h morning stiffness. There is no history of rashes, oral ulcers, fever, Raynaud's phenomenon, or hair loss. She has been taking naproxen 440 mg twice a day with mild benefit. On examination the only significant findings are soft tissue swelling and tenderness of her metacarpal phalangeal joints, wrists, metatarsal phalangeal joints, and knees. There are two-plus effusions of both knees. Rheumatoid factor is strongly positive and antibodies to cyclic citrullinated protein are present. You direct her to remain on naproxen and suggest that she add which of the following drugs?

a. Sulindac
b. Cyclophosphamide
c. Prednisone 60 mg per day for 3 months with subsequent tapering
d. Prednisone 10 mg per day for 2 weeks with subsequent tapering
e. Tetracycline for 2 weeks

DIRECTIONS: Each group of questions below consists of lettered options followed by a set of numbered items. For each numbered item select the **one** lettered option with which it is **most** closely associated. Each lettered option may be used once, more than once, or not at all.

Questions 87–90

Select the most probable diagnosis for each patient.

a. Behçet's syndrome
b. Ankylosing spondylitis
c. Polymyalgia rheumatica
d. Reiter's syndrome
e. Drug-induced lupus erythematosus
f. Polyarteritis nodosa
g. Polymyositis

87. A 50-year-old drug abuser presents with fever and weight loss. Exam shows hypertension, nodular skin rash, and peripheral neuropathy. ESR is 100 mm/L, and RBC casts are seen on urinalysis.

88. An elderly male presents with pain in his shoulders and hips. ESR is 105 mm/L.

89. A young male presents with leg swelling and recurrent aphthous ulcers of his lips and tongue. He has also recently noted painful genital ulcers. There is no urethritis or conjunctivitis. On exam, he has evidence of deep vein thrombophlebitis.

90. A 19-year-old male complains of low back morning stiffness, pain, and limitation of motion of shoulders. He has eye pain and photophobia. Diastolic murmur is present on physical exam.

Questions 91–95

Match each description with the appropriate disease.

a. Microscopic polyangiitis
b. Classic polyarteritis nodosa
c. Giant cell arteritis
d. Multiple cholesterol embolization syndrome
e. Takayasu's arteritis

91. A 55-year-old woman presents with a 2-month history of fever, weight loss, dyspnea, and microscopic hematuria with RBC casts. A lung biopsy demonstrates pulmonary capillaritis.

92. A 78-year-old man undergoes cardiac PTCA. Over the ensuing 2 days he develops ecchymoses and patchy digital and dermal necrosis involving his arms and legs.

93. A 78-year-old man presents with a 2-month history of fever and intermittent abdominal pain. He develops peritoneal signs and at laparotomy is found to have an area of infarcted bowel. Biopsy shows inflammation of small to medium-sized muscular arteries.

94. A 78-year-old man presents with a 2-month history of headaches. He recently noted pain at the angle of his jaws when he chews.

95. A 20-year-old female competitive swimmer notes that her arms now ache after swimming one or two laps, and she is unable to continue. She has had night sweats and a 10-lb weight loss.

Rheumatology

Answers

61. The answer is a. *(Kasper, pp 1972–1973.)* The clinical picture of symmetrical swelling and tenderness of the metacarpophalangeal (MCP) and wrist joints lasting longer than 6 weeks strongly suggests rheumatoid arthritis. Rheumatoid factor, an immunoglobulin directed against the Fc portion of IgG, is positive in about two-thirds of cases and may be present early in the disease. The history of lethargy or fatigue is a common prodrome of RA. The inflammatory joint changes on exam are not consistent with chronic fatigue syndrome; furthermore, patients with CFS typically report fatigue existing for many years. The MCP-wrist distribution of joint symptoms makes osteoarthritis very unlikely. The x-ray changes described are characteristic of RA, but would occur later in the course of the disease. Although arthritis can occasionally be a manifestation of hematologic malignancies and, rarely, other malignancies, the only indicated screening would be a complete history and physical exam along with a CBC.

62. The answer is b. *(Kasper, pp 1972–1976.)* The patient has more than four of the required signs or symptoms of RA, including morning stiffness, swelling of the wrist or MCP, simultaneous swelling of joints on both sides of body, subcutaneous nodules, and positive rheumatoid factor. Subcutaneous nodules and anti-CCP antibodies are poor prognostic signs for the activity of the disease, and disease-modifying antirheumatic drugs (DMARDs) such as gold, antimalarials, sulfasalazine, methotrexate, leflunamide, anti-TNF agents, or a combination of these drugs should be instituted. Methotrexate has emerged as a cornerstone of most disease-modifying regimens, to which other agents are often added. Low-dose corticosteroids have recently been shown to reduce the progression of bony erosions and, although controversial, are considered by some to be appropriate disease-modifying agents for long-term therapy. Use of anti-inflammatory doses of both aspirin and nonsteroidals together is not desirable because it will increase the risk of side effects. Given the aggressive nature of this woman's rheumatoid arthritis and negative prognostic signs, delay in initiating DMARDs is contraindicated. Significant joint damage has been shown by MRI to occur quite early in the course of disease.

63. The answer is b. (*Kasper, pp 1990–1993.*) The complaints described are characteristic of Sjögren syndrome, an autoimmune disease with presenting symptoms of dry eyes and dry mouth. The disease is caused by lymphocytic infiltration and destruction of lacrimal and salivary glands. The Schirmer test, which assesses tear production by measuring the amount of wetness on a piece of filter paper placed in the lower eyelid for 5 min, is the appropriate screening test. Most patients with Sjögren syndrome produce autoantibodies, particularly anti-Ro (SSA). Lip biopsy is needed only to evaluate uncertain cases, such as when dry mouth occurs without dry eye symptoms. Mumps can cause bilateral parotitis, but would not explain the patient's complaint of a gritty sensation, which is the most typical symptom of dry eye syndrome. Corticosteroids are reserved for severe vasculitis or other serious complications. Although anxiety for which a benzodiazepam could be administered can cause a dry mouth, it would not cause either parotid swelling or dry eyes.

64. The answer is b. (*Kasper, pp 2046–2047.*) The sudden onset and severity of this monoarticular arthritis suggests acute gouty arthritis, especially in a patient on diuretic therapy. However, an arthrocentesis is indicated in the first episode to document gout by demonstrating needle-shaped, negatively birefringent crystals and to rule out other diagnoses such as infection. The level of serum uric acid during an episode of acute gouty arthritis may actually fall. Therefore, a normal serum uric acid does not exclude a diagnosis of gout. For most patients with acute gout, NSAIDs are the treatment of choice. Colchicine is also effective but causes nausea and diarrhea. Antibiotics should not be started for suspected septic arthritis before an arthrocentesis is performed. Treatment for hyperuricemia should not be initiated in the setting of an acute attack of gouty arthritis. Long-term goals of management are to control hyperuricemia, prevent further attacks, and prevent joint damage. Long-term prophylaxis with a uricosuric agent or allopurinol is considered for repeated attacks of acute arthritis, urolithiasis, or formation of tophaceous deposits. X-ray of the ankle would likely be inconclusive in this patient with no trauma history. In the absence of evidence of trauma, there is no indication for immobilization.

65. The answer is a. (*Stobo, pp 251–256, Kasper, p 2032.*) The clinical and laboratory picture suggests an acute septic arthritis. The most important first step is to determine the etiologic agent of the infection. Synovial leukocyte counts in gout typically range between 2000/μL and 50,000/μL. There is no history of symptoms suggesting connective tissue disease. Gonococci can cause a septic arthritis, but a urethral culture in the absence of urethral discharge would not be helpful. Antineutrophil cytoplasmic antibodies are present in certain vasculitides. There is no indication of systemic vasculitis in this patient.

66. The answer is d. *(Kasper, pp 818, 2050–2051.)* *S. aureus* is the most common organism to cause septic arthritis in adults. β-hemolytic streptococci are the second most common. *N. gonorrhoeae* can also produce septic arthritis, but would be less likely in this patient who is not sexually active. *S. pneumoniae* and *E. coli* are rare causes of septic arthritis and usually occur secondary to a primary focus of infection. Septic arthritis commonly occurs in joints that are anatomically damaged, such as in this case with prior rheumatoid arthritis. Anytime a patient with arthritis develops a monoarticular flare out of proportion to the rest of the joints, septic arthritis must be suspected.

67. The answer is d. *(Kasper, pp 100–101.)* The patient presents with symptoms consistent with acute mechanical low back pain. Even patients with lumbar disc herniation and sciatica usually improve with nonoperative care, and imaging studies do not affect initial management. Activity as tolerated with optional 2 days of bed rest is recommended along with adequate pain control and reassurance. Active therapy to restore range of motion and function may be appropriate after pain and spasm are relieved.

68. The answer is a. *(Kasper, pp 2036–2045.)* The clinical picture of anarthritis of weight-bearing joints made worse by activity is suggestive of degenerative joint disease, also called osteoarthritis. Osteoarthritis may frequently have a mild to moderate inflammatory component. Crepitation in the involved joints is characteristic, as are bony enlargements of the DIP joints. In this overweight patient, weight reduction is the best method to decrease the risk of further degenerative changes. Aspirin, other NSAIDs, or acetaminophen can be used as symptomatic treatment but do not affect the course of the disease. Calcium supplementation may be relevant to associated osteoporosis, but does not treat osteoarthritis. Oral prednisone would not be indicated. Intraarticular corticosteroid injections may be given two to three times per year for symptom reduction. Glucosamine may provide further symptomic relief. Knee replacement is the treatment of last resort, usually when symptoms are not controlled by medical regimens and/or activities are severely limited.

69. The answer is b. (*Kasper, pp 1993–2001.*) Insidious back pain occurring in a young male that improves with exercise suggests one of the spondyloarthropathies—ankylosing spondylitis, reactive arthritis (including Reiter's syndrome), psoriatic arthritis, or enteropathic arthritis. In the absence of symptoms or findings to suggest one of the other conditions and in the presence of symmetrical sacroiliitis on x-ray, ankylosing spondylitis is the most likely diagnosis. Acute lumbosacral strain would not be relieved by exercise or worsened by rest. The prognosis in ankylosing spondylitis is generally very good, with only 6% dying of the disease itself. While pulmonary fibrosis and restrictive lung disease can occur, they are rarely a cause of death (cervical fracture, heart block, and amyloidosis are leading causes of death due to ankylosing spondylitis). Rheumatoid factor is negative in all the spondyloarthropathies. Crohn's disease can cause an enteropathic arthritis, and the arthritis may precede the gastrointestinal manifestations, but this diagnosis is far less likely in this case than ankylosing spondylitis.

70. The answer is a. (*Kasper, pp 1960–1967.*) The combination of fever, malar rash, and arthritis suggests systemic lupus erythematosus, and the patient's thrombocytopenia, leukopenia, and positive antibody to native DNA provide more than four criteria for a definitive diagnosis. Other criteria for the diagnosis of lupus include discoid rash, photosensitivity, oral ulcers, serositis, renal disorders (proteinuria or cellular casts), and neurologic disorder (seizures). High-dose corticosteroids would be indicated for severe or life-threatening complications of lupus such as described in item a. Patients with SLE have an unpredictable course. Few patients develop all signs or symptoms. Neuropsychiatric disease occurs·at some time in about half of all SLE patients and Raynaud's phenomenon in about 25%. Pregnancy is relatively safe in women with SLE who have controlled disease and are on less than 10 mg of prednisone.

71. The answer is b. (*Kasper, pp 1979–1989.*) The symptoms of Raynaud's phenomenon, arthralgia, and dysphagia point toward the diagnosis of scleroderma. Scleroderma, or systemic sclerosis, is characterized by a systemic vasculopathy of small and medium-sized vessels, excessive collagen deposition in tissues, and an abnormal immune system. It is an uncommon multisystem disease affecting women more often than men. There are two variants of scleroderma—a relatively benign type called the CREST syndrome and a more severe, diffuse disease. Antinucleolar antibody occurs in only 20 to 30% of patients with the disease, but a positive test is highly specific. Cardiac involvement may occur, and an ECG could show heart block or pericardial involvement but is not at all specific. Renal failure can develop insidiously. Rheumatoid factor is nonspecific and present in 20% of patients with scleroderma. Reproduction of Raynaud's phenomena is nonspecific and is not recommended as an office test.

72. The answer is c. (*Kasper, pp 1996–1998.*) Reiter's syndrome is a reactive polyarthritis that develops several weeks after an infection such as nongonococcal urethritis or gastrointestinal infection caused by *Yersinia enterocolitica, Campylobacter jejuni,* or *Salmonella* or *Shigella* species. Reiter's syndrome is characterized as a triad of oligoarticular arthritis, conjunctivitis, and urethritis. The disease is most common among young men and is associated with the histocompatibility antigen, HLA-B27. Circinate balanitis is a painless red rash on the glans penis that occurs in 25 to 40% of patients. Other clinical features may include keratodermia blenorrhagicum (a rash on the palms and soles indistinguishable from papular psoriasis), spondylitis, and myocarditis. ANA and rheumatoid factor are usually negative. Gonorrhea can precipitate Reiter's syndrome, but patients with the disease are culture-negative.

73. The answer is b. (*Kasper, pp 2047–2049, 2057, 2301.*) Pseudogout is part of the spectrum of calcium pyrophosphate deposition disease. It is usually an acute monoarthritis or oligoarthritis caused by calcium pyrophosphate crystals in the joint. Pseudogout may be associated with hemochromatosis. Since the patient has a history of diabetes mellitus and cardiomyopathy, hemochromatosis must be considered. Serum iron saturation should be measured. Ferritin may also be a useful measure of iron stores. Pseudogout has also been associated with hyperparathyroidism. A familial form of the disease has been localized to chromosomes 8q and 5p. Inflammatory bowel disease, Lyme disease, and peptic ulcer disease do not predispose to pseudogout.

74. The answer is a. (*Kasper, pp 2008–2009.*) Headache and transient unilateral visual loss (amaurosis fugax) in this elderly patient with polymyalgia rheumatica (PMR) symptoms suggest a diagnosis of temporal arteritis. The erythrocyte sedimentation rate is high in almost all cases. Temporal arteritis occurs most commonly in patients over the age of 55 and is highly associated with polymyalgia rheumatica. However, only about 25% of patients with PMR have giant cell arteritis. Older patients who complain of diffuse myalgias and joint stiffness, particularly of the shoulders and hips, should be evaluated for PMR with an ESR. Unilateral visual changes or even unilateral visual loss may occur abruptly in patients with temporal arteritis. Biopsy results should not delay initiation of corticosteroid therapy. Biopsies may show vasculitis even after 14 days of glucocorticoid therapy. Delay risks permanent loss of sight. Once an episode of loss of vision occurs, workup must proceed as quickly as possible. Treatment for temporal arteritis requires relatively high doses of steroids, beginning with prednisone at 40 to 60 mg per day for about 1 month with subsequent tapering. Aspirin should be added because it decreases the risks of vascular occlusions but is not sufficient alone. The treatment for polymyalgia rheumatica without concommitant temporal arteritis requires much lower doses of steroids, in the range of 10 to 20 mg per day of prednisone.

75. The answer is d. (*Kasper, pp 1998–1999.*) Psoriatic arthritis can be very aggressive and destructive. The radiographic pencil-in-cup deformity is a characteristic form of joint destruction in this condition. This man has failed conventional DMARD therapy. Cyclophosphamide is used primarily for life- or organ-threatening vasculitis and is not indicated for arthritis alone. Although cyclosporine has been used for psoriatic arthritis with limited success, it is not as good a choice as a TNF blocking agent. TNF blockers have shown dramatic benefit in regard to both the arthritis and the skin disease. Folic acid supplementation helps decrease the risk of some side effects of methotrexate. It does not improve its therapeutic effectiveness. Although low-dose steroids can be appropriate for inflammatory arthritis, doses higher than 10 mg per day should not be given for sustained periods because of the long-term side effects.

76. The answer is c. (*Kasper, pp 2047–2049.*) Acute monoarticular arthritis in association with linear calcification of the cartilage of the knee representing chondrocalcinosis suggests the diagnosis of pseudogout, a form of calcium pyrophosphate dihydrate deposition disease (CPPDD). In its acute manifestation the disease resembles gout. Positively birefringent crystals (looking blue or green when parallel to the axis of the red compensator on a polarizing microscope) can be demonstrated in joint fluid, although careful search is sometimes necessary. Serum uric acid and calcium levels are normal, as is the rheumatoid factor. Pseudogout is about half as common as gout, but becomes more common after age 65. Calcium pyrophosphate dihydrate deposition disease is diagnosed in symptomatic patients by characteristic x-ray findings of crystals in synovial fluid. Pseudogout is treated with NSAIDs, colchicine, or steroids. Arthrocentesis and drainage with intraarticular steroid administration is also an effective treatment. Linear calcifications or chondrocalcinosis are often found in the joints of elderly patients who do not have symptomatic joint problems; such patients do not require treatment.

77. The answer is a. (*Kasper, pp 2055–2057.*) The patient's multiple tender points, associated sleep disturbance, and lack of joint or muscle findings make fibromyalgia a likely diagnosis. Patients with fibromyalgia often report dropping things due to pain and weakness, but objective muscle weakness is not present on exam. The diagnosis hinges on the presence of multiple tender points in the absence of any other disease likely to cause musculoskeletal symptoms. CBC and ESR are characteristically normal. Tricyclic antidepressants may help restore sleep. Aspirin, other anti-inflammatory drugs, and DMARDs are not helpful. Cognitive behavioral therapy and aerobic exercise programs have been partially successful. However, simple stretching/flexibility exercises have not been shown to be helpful. Of note, rheumatoid factors and antinuclear antibodies occur in a small number of normal individuals. They are more frequent in women and increase in frequency with age. It is not uncommon for an individual with fibromyalgia and an incidentally positive RF or ANA to be misdiagnosed as having collagen vascular disease. Therefore, it is necessary to be careful to separate subjective tenderness on exam from objective musculoskeletal findings and to assiduously search for other criteria before diagnosing RA, SLE, or other collagen vascular disease.

78. The answer is c. (*Kasper, p 2036.*) Hip pain may result from fracture, bursitis, arthritis, tumor, or pain referred from the lumbosacral spine. A film of the right hip is mandatory in this patient. Fracture of the hip must be ruled out, particularly in a woman with mental status abnormalities, who may be prone to falls. Elderly women with osteoporosis are most prone to hip fracture. Pain from the hip joint is most often felt in the groin radiating down the anterior thigh. It is important to realize that patients will often complain of "hip" pain when they mean pain in the buttocks or low back. Pain in the buttocks is most often referred pain from the spine.

79. The answer is c. *(Kasper, p 1972.)* Felty's syndrome consists of the triad of rheumatoid arthritis, splenomegaly, and leukopenia. In contrast to the lymphopenia observed in patients who have systemic lupus erythematosus, the leukopenia of Felty's syndrome is related to a reduction in the number of circulating polymorphonuclear leukocytes. The mechanism of the granulocytopenia is poorly understood. Felty's syndrome tends to occur in people who have had active rheumatoid arthritis for a prolonged period. These patients commonly have other systemic features of rheumatoid disease such as nodules, skin ulcerations, the sicca complex, peripheral sensory and motor neuropathy, and arteritic lesions.

80. The answer is d. *(Kasper, pp 1968–1976.)* This patient has rheumatoid arthritis. The presence of rheumatoid factor and anti-CCP antibodies suggests more aggressive disease with a greater likelihood of progressive joint destruction. Therefore, early aggressive treatment with disease modifying drugs is advisable to prevent irreversible joint damage. Drugs used in the treatment of rheumatoid arthritis are broadly classified as pain relievers, which include anti-inflammatory drugs (NSAIDs), acetaminophen, narcotics, and so on, or disease-modifying antirheumatic drugs (DMARDs). She is already taking an NSAID, naproxen, and it would be inappropriate to add a second NSAID, sulindac. Cyclophosphamide and high-dose prednisone are very rarely used in rheumatoid arthritis, and then only for severe or life-threatening vasculitic complications. A short course of tetracycline would be of no benefit. Low-dose prednisone (5 to 10 mg per day) may be very useful in controlling an acute flare-up of arthritis or in controlling the disease while waiting for a remittive agent to begin working. Recent data also have demonstrated that long-term low-dose steroid administration slows progression of joint damage, and some rheumatologists now use it as a DMARD. Low-dose prednisone would be a good initial addition to an NSAID in this patient. Other DMARDs that could be chosen include methotrexate, hydroxychloroquine, leflunamide, sulfasalazine, gold (used uncommonly at present), or a tumor necrosis factor inhibitor. Azathioprine and cyclosporine are less commonly used DMARDs usually reserved for patients who fail first-line DMARDs.

81. The answer is d. *(Kasper, pp 1968–1976.)* The patient's GI bleeding is most likely due to NSAID gastropathy, an extremely common complication. It may occur without associated abdominal symptoms. Although she recently began hydroxychloroquine, that medicine does not cause GI bleeding. Emotional distress causing ulcer disease, lymphoma, and Meckel's diverticulum are all possible, but there is nothing in this case history to suggest them, and they are much rarer than NSAID gastropathy.

82. The answer is c. *(Kasper, pp 1968–1976.)* Etanercept, infliximab, and adalimimab are TNF inhibitors that have been shown to be highly efficacious DMARDs. Suppression of the action of TNF is associated with a significantly increased risk of serious infections, a complication requiring vigilance and timely action by physicians. Although all the other conditions listed as answers to question 94 can cause fever, the managing physician must first suspect and rule out a significant infection as a complication of immunosuppressant therapy.

83. The answer is d. *(Kasper, pp 1993–1995.)* This patient has ankylosing spondylitis (AS), confirmed by typical radiographic features. Traditionally, AS management has been limited to NSAIDs, which provide only mild symptomatic relief. The progression of ankylosing spondylitis resulting in limited mobility or even total spinal rigidity is not impacted by NSAIDs. Physical therapy may help maintain posture as the ankylosis progresses but does not affect the long term progression of the spinal disease. Tumor necrosis factor inhibitors (see above answer) have been demonstrated to be efficacious in AS and offer the best option for limitation of disease progression.

84. The answer is c. *(Kasper, pp 2004–2006.)* Wegener's granulomatosis (WG) is a granulomatous vasculitis of small arteries and veins that affects the lungs, sinuses, nasopharynx, and kidneys, where it causes a focal and segmental glomerulonephritis. Other organs can also be damaged, including the skin, eyes, and nervous system. Most patients with the disease develop antibodies to certain proteins in the cytoplasm of neutrophils called antineutrophil cytoplasmic antibodies (ANCA). The most common ANCA staining pattern seen in WG is cytoplasmic, C-ANCA. A perinuclear pattern, P-ANCA, is sometimes seen. The C-ANCA pattern is usually caused by antibodies to proteinase-3, whereas P-ANCA is usually caused by antibodies to myeloperoxidase. Henoch-Schönlein purpura and classic polyarteritis generally do not involve the upper airways. Sarcoidosis may involve the upper respiratory tract (20%), but it does not cause bloody nasal discharge and does not cause glomerulonephritis.

85. The answer is c. (*Kasper, pp 2055–2057.*) The signs and symptoms suggest fibromyalgia. Fibromyalgia is a very common disorder, particularly in middle-aged women, characterized by diffuse musculoskeletal pain, fatigue, and nonrestorative sleep. The American College of Rheumatology has established diagnostic criteria for the disease, which include a history of widespread pain in association with 11 of 18 specific tender point sites. In this patient with very characteristic signs and symptoms, the identification of 11 specific trigger points would be the best method of diagnosis. Polymyalgia rheumatica may sometimes be in the differential diagnosis. In this patient PMR would be particularly unlikely given the normal ESR. Fibromyalgia is distinct from inflammatory muscle disease like polymyositis or dermatomyositis. Patients with inflammatory muscle disease usually present with proximal muscle weakness and have elevated muscle enzymes, whereas patients with fibromyalgia usually complain predominantly of musculoskeletal pain and have normal muscle enzymes. Muscle pain is less prominent in inflammatory muscle disease. Fibromyalgia has been associated with other somatic syndromes, including irritable bladder, irritable bowel syndrome, headaches, and temporomandibular joint pain. Patients with fibromyalgia have an increased lifetime incidence of psychiatric disorders, particularly depression and panic disorder. However, there is convincing evidence that fibromyalgia is a disease of abnormal central nervous pain processing associated with amplification of nociceptive stimuli. This suggests that the demonstrated lower thresholds for noxious stimuli are due to a CNS abnormality of as yet undetermined etiology. Steroids and NSAIDs have not been shown to be helpful in fibromyalgia and would not be expected to be so since there is no evidence of inflammation.

86. The answer is a. *(Kasper, pp 2501–2502.)* Carpal tunnel syndrome results from median nerve entrapment and is frequently due to excessive use of the wrist. The process has also been associated with thickening of connective tissue, as in acromegaly, or with deposition of amyloid. It also occurs in hypothyroidism, rheumatoid arthritis, and diabetes mellitus. As in this patient, numbness is frequently worse at night and relieved by shaking the hand. Atrophy of the abductor pollicis brevis as evidenced by thenar wasting is a sign of advanced disease and an indication for surgery. Tinel's sign (paresthesia induced in the median nerve distribution by tapping on the volar aspect of the wrist) is very characteristic but not specific. De Quervain's tenosynovitis causes focal wrist pain on the radial aspect of the hand and is due to inflammation of the tendon sheath of the abductor pollicis longus. It should not produce a positive Tinel sign or evidence of median nerve dysfunction. Amyotrophic lateral sclerosis may present with distal muscle weakness but is not usually focal. Diffuse atrophy and muscle fasiculations would be prominent. Rheumatoid arthritis would not produce these symptoms unless inflammation of the wrist was causing median nerve entrapment in the carpal tunnel. Guillain-Barré syndrome is a rapidly progressive polyneuropathy that typically presents with an ascending paralysis.

87–90. The answers are 87-f, 88-c, 89-a, 90-b. *(Kasper, pp 1972, 1993–1995, 2007–2008, 2009.)* The 50-year-old drug abuser has a multisystem disease, including systemic complaints, hypertension, skin lesions, neuropathy, and an abnormal urinary sediment. This complex suggests a vasculitis, particularly classic polyarteritis nodosa. Twenty to 30% of patients have hepatitis B antigenemia. The disease is a necrotizing vasculitis of small and medium muscular arteries. The pathology of the kidney includes an arteritis and, in some cases, a glomerulitis. Nodular skin lesions show vasculitis on biopsy.

The elderly male presents with nonspecific joint complaints typical of polymyalgia rheumatica. The high erythrocyte sedimentation rate is characteristic.

Behçet's syndrome is a multisystem disorder that usually presents with recurrent oral and genital ulcers. One-fourth of patients develop superficial or deep vein thrombophlebitis. Iritis, uveitis, and nondeforming arthritis may also occur.

The 19-year-old with low back pain, morning stiffness, and eye pain has complaints that suggest ankylosing spondylitis. This is an inflammatory disorder that affects the axial skeleton. It has a close association with HLA-B27 histocompatibility antigen. Anterior uveitis is the most common extraarticular complication. Aortic regurgitation and cardiac conduction abnormalities occur in a few percent of patients.

91–95. The answers are 91-a, 92-d, 93-b, 94-c, 95-e. *(Kasper, pp 1706–1707, 2007–2010.)* The 55-year-old woman presents with a multisystem disease including glomerulonephritis. Lung biopsy shows inflammation of capillaries. These findings fulfill the Chapel Hill criteria for microscopic polyarteritis. Microscopic polyarteritis may involve the lungs, whereas classic polyarteritis nodosa rarely does so.

Elderly people may have extensive atherosclerosis. Especially after an endovascular procedure (such as vascular catheterization, grafting, or repair), some of the atheromatous material may embolize, usually to the skin, kidneys, or brain. This material is capable of fixing complement and thus causing vascular damage. The skin lesions—ecchymoses and necrosis—look much like vasculitis. Differentiation between cholesterol embolization and idiopathic vasculitis is important, since not only is the former not steroid-sensitive, but there have been reports of increasing damage after the institution of steroid therapy.

The patient in question 93 has classic polyarteritis nodosa. It is a multisystem necrotizing vasculitis that, prior to the use of steroids and cyclophosphamide, was uniformly fatal. Patients commonly present with signs of vascular insufficiency in the involved organs. Abdominal involvement is common. In 30% of patients, antecedent hepatitis B virus infection can be demonstrated; immune complexes containing the virus have been found in such patients and are likely pathogenetic.

Giant cell arteritis, also referred to as temporal arteritis or cranial arteritis, is a disease that classically affects the temporal arteries in individuals over 50 years of age. Giant cell arteritis, named for the presence of giant cells and granulomata that disrupt the internal elastic lamina of the vessel, may present with headache, unilateral visual symptoms, jaw claudication, anemia, a high ESR (although a normal ESR does not rule out the diagnosis), and occasionally a syndrome known as polymyalgia rheumatica. Polymyalgia rheumatica manifests as stiffness, aching, and tenderness of the proximal muscles of the shoulder and hip girdles. Muscle enzymes are normal. Giant cell arteritis usually responds to steroid therapy with 40 to 60 mg/d of prednisone; polymyalgia rheumatica typically responds to low-dose prednisone at 10 to 15 mg/d.

The female swimmer has Takayasu's arteritis, a granulomatous inflammation of the aorta and its main branches. Symptoms are due to local vascular occlusion. Her symptoms are due to bilateral arm claudication. Systemic symptoms of arthralgia, fatigue, malaise, anorexia, and weight loss may occur and may precede the vascular symptoms. Surgery may be necessary to correct occlusive lesions.

Pulmonary Disease

Questions

DIRECTIONS: Each item below contains a question followed by suggested responses. Select the **one best** response to each question.

96. A 50-year-old patient with long-standing chronic obstructive lung disease develops the insidious onset of aching in the distal extremities, particularly the wrists bilaterally. There is a 10-lb weight loss. The skin over the wrists is warm and erythematous. There is bilateral clubbing. Plain film is read as periosteal thickening, possible osteomyelitis. Which of the following is the most appropriate management of this patient?

a. Start ciprofloxacin
b. Obtain chest x-ray
c. Aspirate both wrists
d. Begin gold therapy
e. Obtain erythrocyte sedimentation rate

97. A patient with low-grade fever and weight loss has poor excursion on the right side of the chest with decreased fremitus, flatness to percussion, and decreased breath sounds all on the right. The trachea is deviated to the left. Which of the following is the most likely diagnosis?

a. Pneumothorax
b. Pleural effusion
c. Consolidated pneumonia
d. Atelectasis
e. Chronic obstructive lung disease

98. A 40-year-old alcoholic develops cough and fever. Chest x-ray shows an air-fluid level in the superior segment of the right lower lobe. Which of the following is the most likely etiologic agent?

a. *Streptococcus pneumoniae*
b. *Haemophilus influenzae*
c. *Legionella*
d. Anaerobes
e. *Mycoplasma pneumoniae*

99. A 30-year-old male is admitted to the hospital after a motorcycle accident that resulted in a fracture of the right femur. The fracture is managed with traction. Three days later the patient becomes confused and tachypneic. A petechial rash is noted over the chest. Lungs are clear to auscultation. Arterial blood gases show P_{O_2} of 50, P_{CO_2} of 28, and pH of 7.49. Which of the following is the most likely diagnosis?

a. Unilateral pulmonary edema
b. Hematoma of the chest
c. Fat embolism
d. Pulmonary embolism
e. Early *Staphylococcus aureus* pneumonia

100. A 70-year-old patient with chronic obstructive lung disease requires 2 L of nasal O_2 to treat his hypoxia, which is sometimes associated with angina. While receiving nasal O_2, the patient develops pleuritic chest pain, fever, and purulent sputum. He becomes stuporous and develops a respiratory acidosis with CO_2 retention and worsening hypoxia. Which of the following is the treatment of choice?

a. Stop oxygen
b. Begin medroxyprogesterone
c. Intubate and begin mechanical ventilation
d. Observe patient 24 h before changing therapy
e. Begin sodium bicarbonate

101. A 34-year-old black female presents to your office with symptoms of cough, dyspnea, and lymphadenopathy. Physical exam shows cervical adenopathy and hepatomegaly. Her chest radiograph is shown below. Which of the following is most likely to aid in establishing a diagnosis?

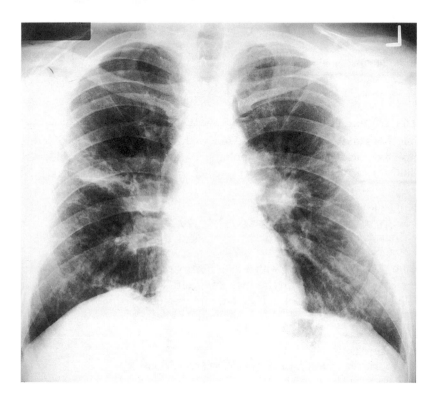

a. Open lung biopsy
b. Liver biopsy
c. Bronchoscopy and transbronchial lung biopsy
d. Scalene node biopsy
e. Serum angiotensin converting enzyme (ACE) level

102. A 64-year-old woman is found to have a left-sided pleural effusion on chest x-ray. Analysis of the pleural fluid reveals a ratio of concentration of total protein in pleural fluid to serum of 0.38, a lactate dehydrogenase (LDH) level of 125 IU, and a ratio of LDH concentration in pleural fluid to serum of 0.46. Which of the following disorders is most likely in this patient?   *Transudate   Protein   Pleural:Serum < .5*
                                                        LDH Pleural:Serum <.6

a. Bronchogenic carcinoma
b. Congestive heart failure
c. Pulmonary embolism
d. Sarcoidosis
e. Systemic lupus erythematosus

103. A 25-year-old male cigarette smoker has a history of respiratory infections and has also been found to have hematuria. A high value for diffusing capacity is noted during pulmonary function testing. This elevated diffusing capacity is consistent with which of the following disorders?

a. Anemia
b. Cystic fibrosis
c. Emphysema
d. Intrapulmonary hemorrhage

104. A 28-year-old male with a long history of severe asthma presents to the emergency room with shortness of breath. He has previously required admission to the hospital and was once intubated for asthma. Which of the following findings on physical exam would indicate a benign course?

a. Silent chest
b. Hypercapnia
c. Thoracoabdominal paradox (paradoxical respiration)
d. Pulsus paradoxus of 5 mmHg
e. Altered mental status

105. A 40-year-old man without a significant past medical history comes to the emergency room with a 3-day history of fever and shaking chills; a 15-min episode of rigor; nonproductive cough; anorexia; and the development of right-sided pleuritic chest pain and shortness of breath over the past 12 h. A chest x-ray reveals a consolidated right middle lobe infiltrate, and a CBC shows an elevated neutrophil count with many band forms present. Which of the following statements regarding pneumonia in this patient is correct?

a. Sputum culture is more helpful than sputum Gram stain in choosing empiric antibiotic therapy
b. If the Gram stain revealed numerous gram-positive diplococci, numerous white blood cells, and few epithelial cells, *Streptococcus pneumoniae* would be the most likely diagnosis
c. Although *S. pneumoniae* is the agent most likely to be the cause of this patient's pneumonia, this diagnosis would be very unlikely if blood cultures were negative
d. The absence of rigors would rule out a diagnosis of pneumococcal pneumonia
e. Penicillin is the drug of choice in all cases of pneumococcal pneumonia

106. A 57-year-old man develops acute shortness of breath shortly after a 12-h automobile ride. The patient is admitted to the hospital for shortness of breath. Findings on physical examination are normal except for tachypnea and tachycardia. An electrocardiogram reveals sinus tachycardia but is otherwise normal. Which of the following statements is correct?

a. A definitive diagnosis can be made by history alone
b. The patient should be admitted to the hospital, and, if there is no contraindication to anticoagulation, intravenous heparin should be started pending further testing
c. Normal findings on examination of the lower extremities are extremely unusual in this clinical setting
d. Early treatment has little effect on overall mortality

107. A 60-year-old male develops acute shortness of breath, tachypnea, and tachycardia while hospitalized for congestive heart failure. On physical exam there is no jugular venous distention and the lungs are clear to auscultation and percussion. There is a loud P_2 sound. Examination of the lower extremities shows no edema or tenderness. Which of the following is the most important diagnostic step?

a. Pulmonary angiogram
b. Ventilation-perfusion scan or chest CT
c. D-dimer assay
d. Venous ultrasound

108. An anxious young woman who is taking birth control pills presents to the emergency room with shortness of breath. The absence of which of the following would make the diagnosis of pulmonary embolus unlikely?

a. Wheezing
b. Pleuritic chest pain
c. Tachypnea
d. Hemoptysis
e. Right-sided S_3 heart sound

109. A 65-year-old male with mild congestive heart failure is to receive total hip replacement. He has no other underlying diseases and no history of hypertension, recent surgery, or bleeding disorder. Which of the following is the best approach to prevention of pulmonary embolus in this patient?

a. Aspirin 75 mg/d
b. Aspirin 325 mg/d
c. Warfarin with INR of 2 to 3 or low-molecular-weight heparin
d. Early ambulation

110. A 30-year-old athlete with asthma is also a cigarette smoker. Which of the following is characteristic of asthma but not other obstructive lung disease?

a. Hyperinflation is present on chest x-ray
b. Airway obstruction is reversible
c. Hypoxia occurs as a consequence of ventilation-perfusion mismatch
d. The FEV_1/FVC ratio is reduced
e. Exacerbation often occurs as a result of an upper respiratory tract infection

111. A 60-year-old male has had a chronic cough for over 5 years with clear sputum production. He has smoked one pack of cigarettes per day for 20 years and continues to do so. X-ray of the chest shows hyperinflation without infiltrates. Arterial blood gases show a pH of 7.38, P_{CO_2} of 40 mmHg, and P_{O_2} of 65 mmHg. Spirometry shows an FEV_1/FVC of 65%. Which of the following is the most important treatment modality for this patient?

a. Oral corticosteroids
b. Home oxygen
c. Broad-spectrum antibiotics
d. Smoking cessation program
e. Predisone orally

112. A 50-year-old male with emphysema and a chest x-ray that has shown apical blebs develops the sudden onset of shortness of breath and left-sided pleuritic chest pain. Pneumothorax is suspected. Which of the following physical examination findings would confirm the diagnosis?

a. Localized wheezes at the left base
b. Hyperresonance of the left chest with decreased breath sounds
c. Increased tactile fremitus on the left side
d. Decreased breath sounds on the left side with deviation of the trachea to the left
e. Dry crackles at both bases

113. A 30-year-old paraplegic male has a long history of urinary tract infection secondary to an indwelling Foley catheter. He develops fever and hypotension requiring hospitalization, fluid therapy, and intravenous antibiotics. He improves, but over 1 week becomes increasingly short of breath and tachypneic. He develops frothy sputum, diffuse rales, and diffuse alveolar infiltrates. There is no fever, jugular venous distention, S_3 gallop, or peripheral or sacral edema. Which of the following is the best approach to a definitive diagnosis in this patient?

a. Blood cultures
.b. CT scan of the chest
c. Pulmonary capillary wedge pressure
d. Ventilation-perfusion scan

114. A 35-year-old female complains of slowly progressive dyspnea. Her history is otherwise unremarkable, and there is no cough, sputum production, pleuritic chest pain, or thrombophlebitis. She has taken appetite suppressants at different times. On physical exam, there is jugular venous distention, a palpable right ventricular lift, and a loud P_2 heart sound. Chest x-ray shows clear lung fields. ECG shows right axis deviation. A perfusion lung scan is normal, with no segmental deficits. Which of the following is the most likely diagnosis?

a. Primary pulmonary hypertension
b. Recurrent pulmonary emboli
c. Cardiac shunt
d. Interstitial lung disease

115. A 40-year-old woman has had increasing fatigue and shortness of breath for years. She is suspected of having pulmonary hypertension based on a chest x-ray that shows right ventricular hypertrophy. Pulmonary embolus is ruled out by spiral CT scan. A right heart catheterization confirms the diagnosis of primary pulmonary hypertension. Which of the following is the best next step in the management of the patient?

a. Acute drug testing with short-acting pulmonary vasodilators
b. High-dose nifedipine
c. Intravenous prostacyclin
d. Lung transplantation

116. A 60-year-old obese male complains of excessive daytime sleepiness. He has been in good health except for mild hypertension. He drinks alcohol in moderation. The patient's wife states that he snores at night and awakens frequently. Examination of the oropharynx is normal. Which of the following studies is most appropriate?

a. EEG to assess stage sleep patterns
b. Ventilation pattern to detect apnea
c. Arterial O_2 saturation
d. Polysomnography to include all of the above

117. An obese 50-year-old woman complains of insomnia, daytime sleepiness, and fatigue. She is found to have recurrent episodes of arterial desaturation—about 30 events per hour—with evidence of obstructive apnea. Which of the following is the treatment of choice for this patient?

a. Nasal continuous positive airway pressure
b. Uvulopalatopharyngoplasty
c. Weight reduction
d. Tracheostomy

118. A 60-year-old male complains of shortness of breath 2 days after a cholecystectomy. There is no fever, chills, sputum production, or pleuritic chest pain. On physical exam temperature is 99°F, pulse is 75, respiratory rate is 20, and blood pressure is 120/70. There are diminished breath sounds and dullness over the left base. Trachea is shifted to the left side. A chest x-ray shows a retrocardiac opacity that silhouettes the left diaphragm. Which of the following is the most likely anatomical problem in this patient?

a. An acute process causing inflammation
b. A left lower lobe mass
c. Diminished lung volume in the left lower lobe, postoperatively
d. Acute bronchospasm caused by surgery

119. A 55-year-old woman with long-standing chronic lung disease and episodes of acute bronchitis complains of increasing sputum production, which is now on a daily basis. Sputum is thick, and daily sputum production has dramatically increased over several months. There are flecks of blood in the sputum. The patient has lost 8 lb. Fever and chills are absent, and sputum cultures have not revealed specific pathogens. Chest x-ray shows increased pulmonary markings and honeycombing in the lower lobes. CT scan shows a signet ring sign with markedly dilated bronchi. Which of the following is the most likely cause of the patient's symptoms?

a. Pulmonary tuberculosis
b. Exacerbation of chronic lung disease
c. Bronchiectasis
d. Anerboic lung abscess
e. Carcinoma of the lung

120. A 20-year-old fireman comes to the emergency room complaining of headache and dizziness after helping to put out a garage fire. He does not complain of shortness of breath, and the arterial blood gas shows a normal partial pressure of oxygen. Which of the following is the best first step in the management of this patient?

a. Begin oxygen therapy
b. Obtain chest x-ray
c. Obtain carboxyhemoglobin level
d. Obtain CT scan

DIRECTIONS: Each group of questions below consists of lettered options followed by a set of numbered items. For each numbered item, select the **one** lettered option with which it is **most** closely associated. Each lettered option may be used once, more than once, or not at all.

Questions 121–125

Match the patient described with the type of pleural effusion

a. A pH less than 7.0, 100% polymorphonuclear leukocytes
b. Right-sided effusion, protein 2.5 g/dL
c. Pleural fluid glucose less than 15 mg/dL
d. Exudate, 100% lymphocytes
e. Bloody effusion
f. Milky appearance

121. A 65-year-old male complains of shortness of breath at night and wakes up at night very short of breath after a few hours of sleep. On physical exam there is neck vein distention and bilateral rales at the bases. A chest x-ray shows a pleural effusion and cardiomegaly.

122. A 50-year-old male has had fever and night sweats. On physical exam there is diffuse lymphadnopathy with palpable cervical, supraclavicular, and axillary nodes. There is a palpable spleen tip. Chest x-ray shows hilar adenopathy and a left pleural effusion.

123. A 40-year-old drug abuser is admitted for fever and chills and is found to have bacterial pneumonia with *Staphlococcus aureus*. The patient does not improve on vancomycin therapy, and a pleural effusion develops while on therapy.

124. A 35-year-old woman has long-standing arthritis with joint deformities of her wrist and hands. She has a history of arthritis in her family. There is a right-sided pleural effusion that is exudative, with 50% lymphocytes and 50% polymorphonuclear leukocytes.

125. A 68-year-old retired construction worker has complained of aching chest pain and shortness of breath with dry cough. There is marked weight loss and anorexia. A chest x-ray shows pleural effusion with pleural thickening

Questions 126–129

Match the chest x-ray letter with the most likely clinical description.

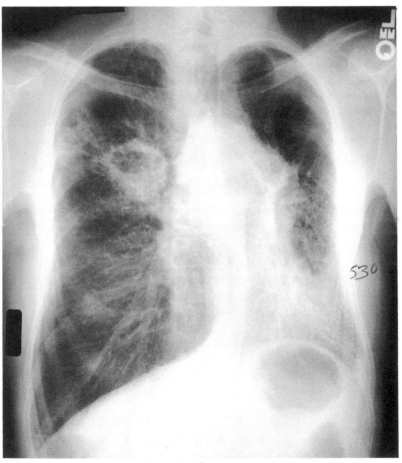

A

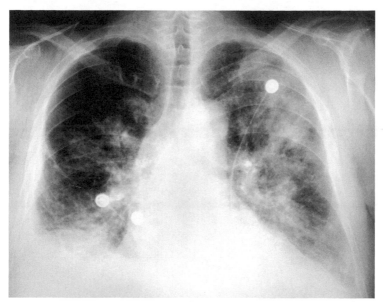

B

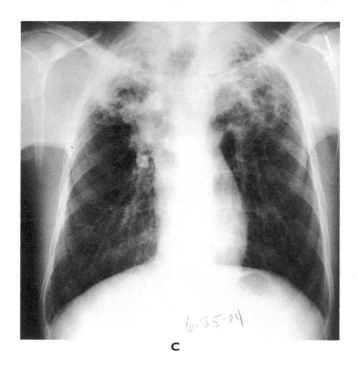

6-25-84

C

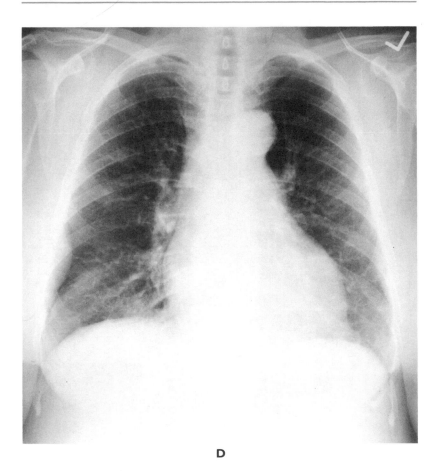

D

126. A 60-year-old has developed fever, chills, and productive cough while in the hospital after surgery. There is increased tactile fremitius at the left base. Sputum Gram stain shows gram-positive cocci in clusters.

127. A 45-year-old male with known coronary artery disease has developed shortness of breath and awakens gasping for breath at night. There is dullness to percussion at the right base.

128. An 85-year-old male, newly arrived from Vietnam, has been complaining of cough and night sweats for more than a year. There are upper lobe crackles bilaterally.

129. A 50-year-old female has had long-standing hypertension that is poorly controlled. Physical exam shows the PMI to be displaced to the sixth intercostal space.

Questions 130–134

For each clinical situation, select the arterial blood gas and pH values with which it is most likely to be associated.

a.   pH 7.50, Po_2 75, Pco_2 28
b.   pH 7.15, Po_2 78, Pco_2 92
c.   pH 7.06, Po_2 36, Pco_2 95
d.   pH 7.06, Po_2 108, Pco_2 13
e.   pH 7.39, Po_2 48, Pco_2 54

130. A 30-year-old obese female bus driver develops sudden pleuritic left-sided chest pain and dyspnea.

131. A 60-year-old heavy smoker has severe chronic bronchitis and peripheral edema and cyanosis.

132. A 22-year-old drug-addicted man is brought to the emergency room by friends who were unable to awaken him.

133. A 62-year-old man who has chronic bronchitis and chest pain is given oxygen via mask in the ambulance en route to the hospital and becomes lethargic in the emergency room.

134. A 20-year-old man with diabetes mellitus comes to the emergency room with diffuse abdominal pain, tachypnea, and fever.

Pulmonary Disease

Answers

96. The answer is b. (*Kasper, pp 2061–2062.*) The clinical picture suggests hypertrophic osteoarthropathy. This process, the pathogenesis of which is unknown, is characterized by clubbing of digits, periosteal new bone formation, and arthritis. Hypertrophic osteoarthropathy is associated with intrathoracic malignancy, suppurative lung disease, and congenital heart problems. Treatment is directed at the underlying disease process. While x-rays may suggest osteomyelitis, the process is usually bilateral and easily distinguishable from osteomyelitis. The first step in evaluation of this patient is to obtain a chest x-ray looking for lung infection and carcinoma.

97. The answer is b. (*Kasper, p 1496.*) The diagnosis in this patient is suggested by the physical exam findings. The findings of poor excursion, flatness of percussion, and decreased fremitus on the right side are all consistent with a right-sided pleural effusion. A large right-sided effusion may shift the trachea to the left. A pneumothorax should result in hyperresonance of the affected side. Atelectasis on the right side would shift the trachea to the right. A consolidated pneumonia would characteristically result in increased fremitus, flatness to percussion, and bronchial breath sounds, and would not cause tracheal deviation.

98. The answer is d. (*Kasper, pp 942–943.*) Of the organisms listed, only anaerobic infection is likely to cause a necrotizing process. *S. pneumoniae* capsular type III pneumococci have been reported to cause cavitary disease, but this is unusual. The location of the infiltrate suggests aspiration, also making anaerobic infection most likely. The superior segment of the right lower lobe is the one most likely to develop an aspiration pneumonia.

99. The answer is c. (*Kasper, p 309.*) Because the clinical signs of neurologic deterioration and a petechial rash have occurred in the setting of fracture and hypoxia, fat embolism is the most likely diagnosis. This process occurs when neutral fat is introduced into the venous circulation after bone trauma or fracture. The latent period is 12 to 36 h. A pulmonary embolus usually has a longer latent period.

100. The answer is c. (*Kasper, pp 1569–1571.*) When stupor and coma supervene in CO_2 retention, fatal arrhythmias, seizures, and death are likely to follow. Stopping oxygen is the worst course of action, as it will exacerbate life-threatening hypoxia. Intubation is the treatment of choice. Bicarbonate plays no role in this acidosis, which is respiratory and caused by hypoventilation.

101. The answer is c. (*Kasper, pp 2017–2022.*) Sarcoidosis is a systemic illness of unknown etiology. There is a higher prevalence in female patients and in the African American population. Many patients have respiratory symptoms, including cough and dyspnea. Hilar and peripheral lymphadenopathy is common, and 20 to 30% of patients have hepatomegaly. The chest x-ray shows symmetrical hilar lymphadenopathy. The diagnostic method of choice is transbronchial biopsy, which will show a mononuclear cell granulomatous inflammatory process. While liver and scalene node biopsies are often positive, noncaseating granulomas are so frequent in these sites that they are not considered acceptable for primary diagnosis. ACE levels are elevated in two-thirds of patients, but false-positive values are common in other granulomatous disease processes.

102. The answer is b. (*Kasper, pp 1565–1567.*) Classifying a pleural effusion as either a transudate or an exudate is useful in identifying the underlying disorder. Pleural fluid is exudative if it has any one of the following three properties: a ratio of concentration of total protein in pleural fluid to serum greater than 0.5, an absolute value of LDH greater than 200 IU, or a ratio of LDH concentration in pleural fluid to serum greater than 0.6. Causes of exudative effusions include malignancy, pulmonary embolism, pneumonia, tuberculosis, abdominal disease, collagen vascular diseases, uremia, Dressler syndrome, and chylothorax. Exudative effusions may also be drug-induced. If none of the aforementioned properties are met, the effusion is a transudate. Differential diagnosis for a transudative effusion includes congestive heart failure, nephrotic syndrome, cirrhosis, Meigs syndrome (benign ovarian neoplasm with effusion), and hydronephrosis.

103. The answer is d. (*Kasper, pp 1502, 1556.*) Carbon monoxide (CO) diffusing capacity provides an estimate of the rate at which oxygen moves by diffusion from alveolar gas to combine with hemoglobin in the red blood cells. It is interpreted as an index of the surface area engaged in alveolar-capillary diffusion. Measurement of diffusing capacity of the lung is done by having the person inspire a low concentration of carbon monoxide. The rate of uptake of the gas by the blood is calculated from the difference between the inspired and expired concentrations. The test can be performed during a single 10-s breath holding or during 1 min of steady-state breathing. The diffusing capacity is defined as the amount of carbon monoxide transferred per minute per millimeter of mercury of driving pressure and correlates with oxygen transport from the alveolus into the capillaries. Primary parenchymal disorders, anemia, and removal of lung tissue decrease the diffusing capacity. Conversely, polycythemia, congestive heart failure, and intrapulmonary hemorrhage tend to increase the value for diffusing capacity. In this patient, the possibility of Goodpasture syndrome would be considered.

104. The answer is d. (*Kasper, p 1511.*) It is extremely important to accurately determine the severity of an exacerbation of asthma, since the major cause of death from asthma is the underestimation of the severity of a particular episode by either the patient or the physician. Silent chest is a particularly ominous finding, because the airway constriction is so great that airflow is insufficient to generate wheezing. Hypercapnia and thoracoabdominal paradox are almost always indicative of exhaustion and respiratory muscle failure or fatigue and generally need to be aggressively treated with mechanical ventilation. Altered mental status is frequently seen with severe hypoxia or hypercapnia, and ventilatory support is usually required. An increased pulsus paradoxus may also be a sign of severe asthma, as it increases with greater respiratory effort and generation of more negative intrathoracic pressures during inspiration. However, a pulsus paradoxus of up to 8 to 10 mmHg is considered normal; thus, a value of 5 mmHg would not be indicative of a severe episode of asthma.

105. The answer is b. (*Kasper, pp 809, 1533.*) Pneumonia is a common disorder and is a major cause of death, particularly in hospitalized elderly patients. Before choosing empiric therapy for presumed pneumonia, it is necessary to know the age of the patient, whether the infection is community-acquired or nosocomial, and whether there are any underlying debilitating illnesses. Community-acquired pneumonias in patients over the age of 35 are most likely due to *S. pneumoniae, Legionella* species (e.g., *pneumophila*), other atypical agents such as *Mycoplasma pneumoniae* and *Chlamydia pneumoniae, Moraxella catarrhalis,* and *Haemophilus influenzae.* In the case outlined, the history is strongly consistent with pneumococcal pneumonia, manifested by a short prodrome, shaking chills with rigor, fever, chest pain, sparse sputum production associated with cough, and a consolidated lobar infiltrate on chest x-ray. The most reliable method of diagnosing pneumococcal pneumonia is seeing gram-positive diplococci on an adequate sputum (many white cells, few epithelial cells). Sputum culture is also important in the era of penicillin-resistant pneumococci, but is not helpful in initial diagnosis. Blood cultures are positive in only about 20% of patients, and, when positive, are indicative of a more severe case. Although rigors may suggest pneumococcal bacteremia, the absence of rigors does not rule out the diagnosis. About 25 to 50% of pneumococci in the United States are partially or completely resistant to penicillin due to chromosomal mutations resulting in penicillin-binding protein changes. Penicillin is no longer the regimen of choice for pneumococcal pneumonia pending the results of sensitivity testing. The fluoroquinolones or ceftriaxone are widely used as initial therapy for pneumococcal pneumonia.

106. The answer is b. (*Kasper, pp 1561–1565.*) The clinical situation described is characteristic of pulmonary embolic disease. In greater than 80% of cases, pulmonary emboli arise from thromboses in the deep venous circulation (DVTs) of the lower extremities. DVTs often begin in the calf, where they rarely if ever cause clinically significant pulmonary embolic disease. However, thromboses that begin below the knee frequently "grow," or propagate, above the knee; clots that dislodge from above the knee cause clinically significant pulmonary emboli, which, if untreated, cause mortality exceeding 80%. Interestingly, only about 50% of patients with DVT of the lower extremities have clinical findings of swelling, warmth, erythema, pain, or "cords." As long as the superficial venous system, which has connections with the deep venous system, remains patent, none of the classic clinical findings of DVT will occur, because blood will drain from the unobstructed superficial system. When a clot does dislodge from the deep venous system and travels into the pulmonary vasculature, the most common clinical findings are tachypnea and tachycardia; chest pain is less likely and is more indicative of concomitant pulmonary infarction. The ABG is usually abnormal, and a high percentage of patients exhibit hypoxia, hypocapnia, alkalosis, and a widening of the alveolar-arterial gradient. The ECG is frequently abnormal in pulmonary embolic disease. The most common finding is sinus tachycardia, but atrial fibrillation, pseudoinfarction in the inferior leads, and right and left axis deviation are also occasionally seen. Initial treatment for suspected pulmonary embolic disease includes prompt hospitalization and institution of intravenous heparin, provided there are no contraindications to anticoagulation. It is particularly important to make an early diagnosis of pulmonary embolus, as intervention can decrease the mortality rate from 25% down to 5%.

107. The answer is b. *(Kasper, pp 1562–1563.)* CT with intravenous contrast is surpassing the ventilation-perfusion scan as a diagnostic method of choice. New multislice scanners can detect central as well as peripheral lesions. Lung scanning is still a useful imaging test for the diagnosis of pulmonary embolus. The diagnosis is very unlikely in patients with normal or near-normal scans, and is highly likely in patients with high-probability scans. In patients with a high clinical index of suspicion for pulmonary embolus but low-probability scan, the diagnosis becomes more difficult, and pulmonary angiography may be indicated. About two-thirds of patients with pulmonary embolus have evidence of deep venous disease on venous ultrasound. Therefore, pulmonary embolus cannot be excluded by a normal study. The quantitative D-dimer enzyme-linked immunoabsorbent assay is positive in 90% of patients with pulmonary embolus in some studies. It has been used to rule out pulmonary embolus in patients with a low- or intermediate-probability scan.

108. The answer is c. *(Kasper, p 1561.)* While all of these signs and symptoms can occur in acute pulmonary embolus, tachypnea is by far the most common. Tachypnea occurs in more than 90% of patients with pulmonary embolus. Pleuritic chest pain occurs in about half of patients and is less common in the elderly and those with underlying heart disease. Hemoptysis and wheezing occur in less than half of patients. A right-sided S_3 is associated with large emboli that result in acute pulmonary hypertension.

109. The answer is c. *(Kasper, p 1565.)* Warfarin is recommended for the prophylaxis of acute pulmonary embolus in patients who receive total hip replacement. Warfarin is started preoperatively, and the daily dose is adjusted to maintain an international normalized ratio (INR) of 2 to 2.5.

Low-molecular-weight heparin given twice daily subcutaneously is also a recommended regimen. The value of aspirin in this setting is unclear. Early ambulation and elastic stockings are also important in preventing thromboembolism, but are not adequate in themselves in this high-risk situation.

110. The answer is b. (*Kasper, p 1511.*) Asthma is an incompletely understood inflammatory process that involves the lower airways and results in bronchoconstriction and excess production of mucus, which in turn lead to increased airway resistance and occasionally respiratory failure and death. During acute exacerbations of asthma, and in other obstructive lung diseases such as chronic obstructive pulmonary disease, hyperinflation may be present on chest x-ray. Hypoxia is common and usually a result of ventilation-perfusion mismatch. The FEV_1/FVC is reduced, and exacerbations are frequently precipitated by upper airway infections. Only in asthma is the airway obstruction reversible.

111. The answer is d. (*Kasper, p 1552.*) This patient's chronic cough, hyperinflated lung fields, abnormal pulmonary function tests, and smoking history are all consistent with chronic bronchitis. A smoking cessation program can decrease the rate of lung deterioration and is successful in as many as 40% of patients, particularly when the physician gives a strong antismoking message and uses both counseling and nicotine replacement. Continuous low-flow oxygen becomes beneficial when arterial oxygen concentration falls below 55 mmHg. Antibiotics are indicated only for acute exacerbations of chronic lung disease, which might present with fever, change in color of sputum, and increasing shortness of breath. Oral corticosteroids are helpful in some patients, but are reserved for those who have failed inhaled bronchodilator treatments.

112. The answer is b. (*Kasper, p 1496.*) The most characteristic findings of pneumothorax are hyperresonance and decreased breath sounds. A tension pneumothorax may displace the mediastinum to the unaffected side. Tactile fremitus would be decreased in the patient with a pneumothorax, but would be increased in conditions in which consolidation of the lung has developed.

113. The answer is c. (*Kasper, pp 1523–1526.*) Sepsis is the most important single cause of adult respiratory distress syndrome. Early in the course of ARDS, patients may appear stable without respiratory symptoms. Tachypnea, hypoxemia, and diffuse infiltrates gradually develop. It may be difficult to distinguish the process from cardiogenic pulmonary edema, especially in patients who have been given large quantities of fluid. This young patient with no evidence of volume overload would be strongly suspected of having ARDS. The pulmonary capillary wedge pressure would be normal or low in ARDS, but elevated in left ventricular failure. ARDS is a complication of sepsis, but blood cultures may or may not be positive. Neither CT of the chest nor ventilation-perfusion scan would be specific enough to help in diagnosis of ARDS.

114. The answer is a. (*Kasper, pp 1405–1406.*) Although a difficult diagnosis to make, primary pulmonary hypertension is the most likely diagnosis in this young woman who has used appetite suppressants. Primary pulmonary hypertension in the United States was associated with fenfluramines. The predominant symptom is dyspnea, which is usually not apparent in the previously healthy young woman until the disease has advanced. When signs of pulmonary hypertension are apparent from physical findings, chest x-ray, or echocardiography, the diagnosis of recurrent pulmonary embolus must be ruled out. In this case, a normal perfusion lung scan makes pulmonary angiography unnecessary. Restrictive lung disease should be ruled out with pulmonary function testing. An echocardiogram will show right ventricular enlargement and a reduction in the left ventricle size consistent with right ventricular pressure overload.

115. The answer is a. (*Kasper, p 1405.*) In all patients in whom primary pulmonary hypertension is confirmed, acute drug testing with a pulmonary vasodilator is necessary to assess the extent of pulmonary vascular reactivity. Inhaled nitric oxide, intravenous adenosine, or intravenous prostacyclin have all been used. Patients who have a good response to the short-acting vasodilator are tried on a long-acting calcium channel antagonist under direct hemodynamic monitoring. Prostacyclin given via the pulmonary artery through a right heart catheterization has been approved for patients who are functional class III or IV and have not responded to calcium channel antagonists. Treprostinil, a prostacyclin and bosentan, an endothelial receptor antagonist have also recently been approved for class III and IV disease. Lung transplantation is reserved for late stages of the disease when patients are unresponsive to prostacyclin. The disease does not appear to recur after transplantation.

116. The answer is d. (*Kasper, pp 1573–1576.*) With the history of daytime sleepiness and snoring at night, the patient requires evaluation for obstructive sleep apnea syndrome. Frequent awakenings are actually more suggestive of central sleep apnea. Polysomnography is required to assess which type of sleep apnea syndrome is present. EEG variables are recorded that identify various stages of sleep. Arterial oxygen saturation is monitored by finger or ear oximetry. Heart rate is monitored. The respiratory pattern is monitored to detect apnea and whether it is central or obstructive. Ambulatory sleep monitoring with oxygen saturation studies alone might identify multiple episodes of desaturation, but negative results would not rule out a sleep apnea syndrome. Overnight oximetry alone can be used in some patients when the index of suspicion for obstructive sleep apnea is high.

117. The answer is a. (*Kasper, pp 1573–1576.*) In this patient with multiple episodes of desaturation, continuous positive airway pressure would be the recommended therapy. Weight loss is often helpful and should be recommended as well, but would probably not be sufficient. Uvulopalatopharyngoplasty has also been used in obstructive sleep apnea, but when applied to unselected patients is effective in less than 50%. Tracheostomy is a course of last resort that does provide immediate relief.

118. The answer is c. (*Kasper, p 43.*) Postoperative atelectasis or volume loss is a very common complication of surgery. General anesthesia and surgical manipulation lead to atelectasis by causing diagraphmatic immobilization. Atelectases is usually basilar. On physical exam, shift of the trachea to the affected side suggests volume loss. On chest x-ray in this patient, loss of the left hemidiaphragm, increased density, and shift of the hilum downward would all suggest left lower lobe collapse. Atelectasis needs to be distinguished from acute consolidation of pneumonia, in which case fever, chills, and purulent sputum are more pronounced and consolidation is present without volume loss.

119. The answer is c. (*Kasper, p 1541.*) While symptoms such as sputum production and cough are nonspecific, particularly in a patient with known chronic lung disease, the high volume of daily sputum production suggests bronchiectasis. In this process, an abnormal and permanent dilatation of bronchi occurs as the muscular and elastic components of the bronchi are damaged. Clearance of secretions becomes a major problem contributing to a cycle of bronchial inflammation and further deterioration. A high-resolution CT scan, now the diagnosis of choice for this disease, shows prominent dilated bronchi and the signet ring sign of dilated bronchus adjacent to pulmonary artery. The specific CT scan picture is pathognomonic for bronchiectasis and makes the diagnosis of lung abscess or tuberculosis unlikely. The increased amount of sputum produced is also very characteristic of bronchiectasis.

120. The answer is c. (*Kasper, pp 1634–1635.*) With symptoms of headache and dizziness in a fireman, the diagnosis of carbon monoxide poisoning must be addressed quickly. A venous or arterial measure of carboxyhemoglobin must first be obtained, if possible, before oxygen therapy is begun. The use of supplementary oxygen prior to obtaining the test may be a confounding factor in interpreting blood levels. Oxygen or even hyperbaric oxygen is given after blood for carboxyhemoglobin is drawn. Chest x-ray should also be obtained. It may be normal or show a pattern of nonpulmonary edema, or aspiration in severe cases. Central nervous system imaging would not be indicated, and there are no diagnostic patterns that are specific to carbon monoxide poisoning.

121–125. The answers are 121-b, 122-d, 123-a, 124-c, 125-e. (*Kasper, pp 1565–1567.*) The first step in determining the cause of a pleural effusion is to categorize it as either a transudate or exudate. Transudative effusions occur when factors alter the formation or absorption of pleural fluid; exudative effusions occur when local factors produce an inflammatory process. Exudative effusions have one of the following characteristics: pleural fluid protein–to–serum protein ratio greater than 0.5, pleural fluid LDH–to–serum LDH ratio greater than 0.6, or pleural fluid LDH more than two-thirds the normal upper limit for serum.

The 65-year-old male with shortness of breath and paroxysmal nocturnal dyspnea has congestive heart failure. CHF usually produces a right-sided pleural effusion. Of all the disease processes listed, it is the only one that results in a transudative effusion.

The 50-year-old male with fever, night sweats, weight loss, and lymphadenopathy requires evaluation for lymphoma. The effusion produced in lymphoma is exudative and lymphocytic. Other abnormalities are often present on chest x-ray, such as mediastinal lymphadenopathy.

The drug abuser with pneumonia has developed empyema, bacterial infection of the pleural space. Empyema may be defined by the very low pH value. It is an exudative effusion with a polymorphonuclear leukocyte predominance. A drainage procedure is usually necessary when the pleural fluid pH is below 7.20, when there is gross pus, or when the fluid shows a positive Gram stain or culture.

The 35-year-old woman has rheumatoid arthritis with rheumatoid lung disease. Rheumatoid effusions are often exudative and may be lymphocytic, but they are best characterized by their very low glucose levels. Pleural fluid glucose levels below 60 mg/dL also occur in malignancy and bacterial infections.

The 68-year-old retired construction worker presents with characteristic features of mesothelioma. Mesotheliomas are primary tumors that arise from mesothelial cells that line the pleural cavity. They produce a very bloody effusion. Thoracoscopy or open pleural biopsy are often necessary to make a definitive diagnosis.

126–129. The answers are 126-a, 127-b, 128-c, 129-d. *(Kasper, pp 818, 956, 1497–1498.)* The 60-year-old male has developed nosocomial pneumonia. A sputum Gram stain showing gram-positive cocci in clusters will grow *Staphylococcus aureus*. Chest x-ray A shows a necrotizing pneumonia characteristic of this infection. Cavities develop in association with lung infection when necrotic lung tissue is discharged into airways. Cavities greater than 2 cm are described as lung abscesses.

The 45-year-old with shortness of breath and paroxysmal nocturnal dyspnea has symptoms suggesting congestive heart failure. Chest x-ray B shows signs of congestive heart failure, including cardiomegaly, bilateral infiltrates, and cephalization. When there has been long-standing venous hypertension, upper lobe vessels become more prominent due to redistribution of pulmonary blood flow. When pulmonary edema becomes severe, fluid extends out from the hila in a bat-wing distribution.

Chest x-ray C is best matched with the Vietnamese patient who has fever and night sweats. This x-ray shows characteristic changes of tubercu-

nodule greater than 3 cm is most often malignant, and the shaggy border of the lesion also suggests malignancy.

Asbestosis is a risk factor for those such as construction workers, shipbuilders, and plumbers who may have long-standing history of direct exposure to asbestos-containing materials. Symptoms are usually subtle and include an annoying dry cough and dyspnea on exertion. Asbestosis on chest x-ray produces a diffuse linear interstitial process at the lung bases. Pleural fibrosis and pleural plaques may also be noted, especially on CT scan.

Cardiology

Questions

DIRECTIONS: Each item below contains a question followed by suggested responses. Select the **one best** response to each question.

143. A 60-year-old male patient on aspirin, an angiotensin-converting enzyme inhibitor, nitrates, and a beta blocker, who is being followed for chronic stable angina, presents to the ER with a history of two or three episodes of more severe and long-lasting anginal chest pain each day over the past 3 days. His ECG and cardiac enzymes are normal. Which of the following is the best course of action?

a. Admit the patient and begin intravenous digoxin
b. Admit the patient and begin intravenous heparin
c. Admit the patient and give prophylactic thrombolytic therapy
d. Admit the patient for observation with no change in medication
e. Increase the doses of current medications and follow closely as an outpatient

144. A 60-year-old white female presents with epigastric pain, nausea and vomiting, heart rate of 50, and pronounced first-degree AV block on ER cardiac monitor. Blood pressure is 130/80. Which of the following coronary arteries is most likely to be involved in this process?

a. Right coronary
b. Left main
c. Left anterior descending
d. Circumflex

145. You are seeing in your office a patient with the chief complaint of relatively sudden onset of shortness of breath and weakness, but no chest pain. ECG shows nonspecific ST-T changes. You should be particularly attuned to the possibility of painless, or silent, myocardial infarction in which of the following patients?

a. Unstable angina patient on multiple medications
b. Elderly diabetic
c. Premenopausal female
d. Inferior MI patient
e. MI patient with PVCs

146. A 45-year-old white female smoker is admitted to the hospital for observation after presenting to the emergency department with vague chest pain. There is no past history of cardiac disease, diabetes, hypertension, or hyperlipidemia. Later that night while in bed she has a recurrence of pain, at which time cardiac monitoring shows a transient elevation of precordial ST segments. The pain is promptly relieved by sublingual nitroglycerin. Physical exam is unremarkable. Which of the following is the best follow-up management plan?

a. Echocardiography and anti-inflammatory therapy
b. EGD and proton pump inhibitor therapy
c. Exercise stress testing; treatment depending on results
d. Coronary angiography; likely treatment with nitrates and calcium channel blockers
e. Chest CT scan; likely treatment with IV heparin

147. Two weeks after hospital discharge for documented myocardial infarction, a 65-year-old returns to your office very concerned about low-grade fever and pleuritic chest pain. There is no associated shortness of breath. Lungs are clear to auscultation and heart exam is free of significant murmurs, gallops, or rubs. ECG is unchanged from the last one in the hospital. Which of the following therapies is likely to be most effective?

a. Antibiotics
b. Anticoagulation with warfarin (Coumadin)
c. An anti-inflammatory agent
d. An increase in antianginal medication
e. An antianxiety agent

148. A 72-year-old male presents to the ER with the chief complaint of shortness of breath that awakens him at night. Physical exam findings include bilateral basilar rales, an S_3 gallop, and evidence of cardiomegaly, all major criteria for the diagnosis of congestive heart failure under the Framingham system. While patients with CHF may display a wide range of symptoms and signs, which of the following are also considered among the major criteria (i.e., more specific to CHF)?

a. Dyspnea on exertion and night cough
b. Right-sided pleural effusion plus hepatomegaly
c. Tachycardia (rate 120 or greater) with new onset or increase in ectopy
d. Neck vein distention and positive hepatojugular reflux
e. Extremity edema and weight gain greater than 2 kg over 1 week

149. A 55-year-old patient presents to you with a history of having recently had a 3-day hospital stay for gradually increasing shortness of breath and leg swelling while away on a business trip. He reports being told he had congestive heart failure then, but is asymptomatic now, with normal vital signs and physical exam. An echocardiogram is obtained that estimates an ejection fraction of 38%. The patient likes to keep medications to a minimum. He is currently on just aspirin plus a statin. Other than remaining on those, which of the following would be the most appropriate medication recommendation at this time?

a. Begin an ACE inhibitor and then add a beta blocker on a scheduled basis
b. Begin digoxin plus furosemide (Lasix) on a scheduled basis
c. Begin spironolactone on a scheduled basis
d. Begin hydralazine plus nitrates on a scheduled basis
e. Just use furosemide (Lasix) plus nitroglycerin if shortness of breath and swelling recur
f. Given his preferences, since he is doing well, no other medication is needed

150. A 32-year-old female is referred to you from an OB-GYN colleague due to the onset of extreme fatigue and dyspnea on exertion 1 month after her second vaginal delivery. By history, physical exam, and echocardiogram, which shows systolic dysfunction, you make the diagnosis of peripartum (postpartum) cardiomyopathy. Which of the following statements is correct?

a. Postpartum cardiomyopathy may occur unexpectedly years after pregnancy and delivery
b. About half of all such patients will recover completely
c. The condition is idiosyncratic; the risk of recurrence in a future pregnancy is no greater than average
d. The postpartum state will require a different therapeutic approach than typical dilated cardiomyopathies

151. Yesterday you admitted a 55-year-old white male to the hospital for an episode of chest pain, and you are seeking to rule out MI plus assess for any underlying coronary artery disease. The patient tends to be anxious about his health. On admission, his lungs were clear, but his heart revealed a grade 1/6 early systolic murmur at the upper left sternal border without radiation. Blood pressure readings have consistently been in the 140/90 to 150/100 range. Serial cardiac enzymes are normal, and resting ECGs have shown no change from the initial finding of left ventricular hypertrophy with secondary ST-T changes ("LVH with strain"). The thought of performing a routine Bruce protocol treadmill exercise test (stress test) comes to mind, but is rejected, primarily due to which of the following?

a. Anticipated difficulty with the patient's anxiety (i.e., he might falsely claim chest pain during the test)
b. The increased risk associated with these high blood pressure readings
c. Concern about the heart murmur, a relative contraindication to stress testing
d. The presence of LVH with ST-T changes on baseline ECG
e. Concern that this represents the onset of unstable angina with unacceptable risk of MI with stress testing

152. A 75-year-old patient presents to the ER after a sudden syncopal episode. He is again alert and in retrospect describes occasional substernal chest pressure and shortness of breath on exertion. His lungs have a few bibasilar rales, and his blood pressure is 110/80. Which of the following classic findings should you expect to hear on cardiac auscultation?

a. A harsh systolic crescendo-decrescendo murmur heard best at the upper right sternal border
b. A diastolic decrescendo murmur heard at the mid-left sternal border
c. A holosystolic murmur heard best at the apex
d. A midsystolic click

153. A 72-year-old male comes to the office with intermittent symptoms of dyspnea on exertion, palpitations, and cough occasionally productive of blood. On cardiac auscultation, a low-pitched diastolic rumbling murmur is faintly heard toward the apex. The origin of the patient's problem probably relates to which of the following?

a. Rheumatic fever as a youth
b. Long-standing hypertension
c. A silent MI within the past year
d. A congenital condition

154. You are helping with school sports physicals and see a 13-year-old boy who has had some trouble keeping up with his peers. He has a cardiac murmur, which you correctly diagnose as a ventricular septal defect based on which of the following auscultatory findings?

a. A systolic crescendo-decrescendo murmur heard best at the upper right sternal border with radiation to the carotids; the murmur is augmented with transient exercise
b. A systolic murmur at the pulmonic area and a diastolic rumble along the left sternal border
c. A holosystolic murmur at the mid-left sternal border
d. A diastolic decrescendo murmur at the mid-left sternal border
e. A continuous murmur through systole and diastole at the upper left sternal border

155. A 40-year-old male in generally good health presents to the office with a history of palpitations that last for a few seconds and occur two or three times a week. There are no other symptoms. ECG shows a rare single unifocal premature ventricular contraction (PVC). Which of the following is the most likely cause of this finding?

a. Underlying coronary artery disease
b. Valvular heart disease
c. Hypertension
d. Apathetic hyperthyroidism
e. Idiopathic or unknown

156. A 30-year-old female presents with a chief complaint of palpitations. A 24-h Holter monitor is obtained and shows occasional unifocal PVCs and premature atrial contractions. Which of the following is the best antiarrhythmic management in this patient?

a. Anxiolytic therapy
b. Beta blocker therapy
c. Digoxin
d. Quinidine
e. Reassurance, no medication

157. An active 78-year-old female has been followed for hypertension but presents with new onset of mild left hemiparesis and the finding of atrial fibrillation on ECG, which persists throughout the hospital stay. She had been in sinus rhythm on checkup 3 months earlier. Optimal management by the time of hospital discharge includes review of antihypertensive therapy, a ventricular rate control agent if needed, plus which of the following?

a.   Automated implanted cardioverter-defibrillator (AICD)/permanent pacemaker placement to avoid the need for anticoagulation
b.   Waiting for anticoagulation therapy until the ability to ambulate without falls is established
c.   Antiplatelet therapy such as aspirin, without warfarin (Coumadin)
d.   Warfarin (Coumadin) with a target INR of 1.5 plus antiplatelet therapy
e.   Warfarin (Coumadin) with a target INR of 2.5

158. A 36-year-old white female nurse comes to the ER due to a sensation of fast heart rate, slight dizziness, and vague chest fullness. Blood pressure is 110/70. The following rhythm strip is obtained, which shows which of the following?

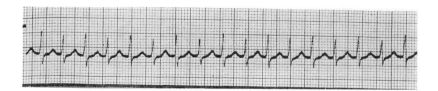

a. Atrial fibrillation
b. Atrial flutter
c. Supraventricular tachycardia
d. Ventricular tachycardia

159. During a new-patient history and physical exam this asymptomatic 67-year-old male was found to have a palpable, pulsatile, but nontender abdominal mass just above the umbilicus. On follow-up ultrasound, an infrarenal abdominal aortic aneurysm is confirmed, measuring 3.0×3.5 cm. The patient's other medical conditions include hypertension, hyperlipidemia, and tobacco abuse. Which of the following is an accurate, evidence-based recommendation for the patient to consider?

a. Watchful waiting is the best course until the first onset of abdominal pain
b. Surgery would be indicated except for the excess operative risk represented by the patient's risk factors
c. Serial follow-up with ultrasound, CT, or MRI is indicated, with the major determinant for surgery being aneurysmal size greater than 5 to 6 cm
d. Serial follow-up with ultrasound, CT, or MRI is indicated, with the major determinant for surgery being involvement of a renal artery
e. Unlike stents in the setting of coronary artery disease, endovascular stent grafts have proven unsuccessful in the management of AAAs

160. A 65-year-old man with diabetes, on an oral hypoglycemic, presents to the ER with a sports-related right shoulder injury. His heart rate was noted to be irregular, and the following ECG was obtained. Which of the following is the best immediate therapy?

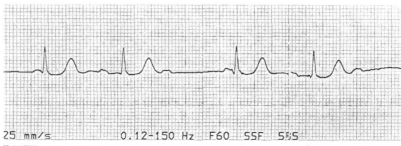

a. Atropine
b. Isoproterenol
c. Pacemaker placement
d. Electrical cardioversion
e. Digoxin
f. Diltiazem
g. Observation

161. In the ICU, a patient suddenly becomes unresponsive, pulseless, and hypotensive, with cardiac monitor indicating ventricular tachycardia. The crash cart is immediately available. The first therapeutic step should be?

a. Amiodarone 150 mg IV push
b. Lidocaine 1.5 mg/kg IV push
c. Epinephrine 1 mg IV push
d. Defibrillation at 200 joules
e. Defibrillation at 360 joules

162. A 70-year-old female has been relatively healthy (but allergic to penicillin), treated only for hypertension, on a thiazide diuretic. She comes to the hospital due to the sudden onset of a severe, tearing chest pain, which radiates through to the back, associated with dyspnea and diaphoresis. Blood pressure is 165/80. Lung auscultation reveals bilateral basilar rales. A faint murmur of aortic insufficiency is heard. The BNP level is elevated at 550 pg/mL. ECG shows nonspecific ST-T changes. A chest x-ray suggests a widened mediastinum. Which of the following choices represents the most prudent emergent management?

a. IV furosemide plus IV loading dose of digoxin
b. Emergent percutaneous coronary intervention with consideration of angioplasty and/or stenting
c. Blood cultures followed by rapid initiation of vancomycin plus gentamicin, then echocardiography
d. IV beta-blocker therapy plus echocardiography; consideration of nitroprusside
e. IV heparin followed by chest CT scan; consideration of thrombolytic therapy

163. A 55-year-old African American female presents to the ER with lethargy and blood pressure of 250/150. Her family members indicate that she was complaining of severe headache and visual disturbance earlier in the day. They report a past history of asthma but no known kidney disease. On physical exam, retinal hemorrhages are present. Which of the following is the best approach?

a. Intravenous labetalol therapy
b. Continuous-infusion nitroprusside
c. Clonidine by mouth to lower blood pressure slowly but surely
d. Nifedipine sublingually to lower blood pressure rapidly
e. Further history about recent home antihypertensives before deciding current therapy

164. An 18-year-old male complains of fever and transient pain in both knees and elbows. The right knee was red and swollen for 1 day during the week prior to presentation. On physical exam, the patient has a low-grade fever but appears generally well. There is a diastolic murmur heard at the base of the heart. A nodule is palpated over an extensor tendon of the hand. There are pink erythematous lesions over the abdomen, some with central clearing. The following laboratory values are obtained:

CBC:
Hct: 42
WBC: 12,000/μL with 80% polymorphonuclear leukocytes, 20% lymphocytes
ESR: 60 mm/h

The patient's ECG is shown below. Which of the following tests is most critical to diagnosis?

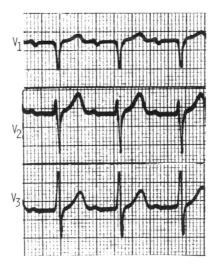

a. Blood cultures
b. Antistreptolysin O antibody
c. Echocardiogram
d. Antinuclear antibodies
e. Creatinine phosphokinase

165. A 36-year-old male comes with the sensation of a racing heart. His blood pressure is 110/70, respiratory rate normal, and O_2 saturation 98%. His ECG shows a narrow QRS complex tachycardia with rate 180, which you correctly diagnose as paroxysmal atrial tachycardia. Which of the following is the initial therapy of choice in this hemodynamically stable patient?

a. Adenosine 6 mg rapid IV bolus
b. Verapamil 2.5 to 5 mg IV over 1 to 2 min
c. Diltiazem 0.25 mg/kg IV over 2 min
d. Digoxin 0.5 mg IV slowly
e. Lidocaine 1.5 mg/kg IV bolus
f. Electrical cardioversion at 50 joules

166. A patient has been in the coronary care unit for the past 24 h with an acute anterior myocardial infarction. He develops the abnormal rhythm shown below, although blood pressure remains stable at 110/68. Which of the following is the best next step in therapy?

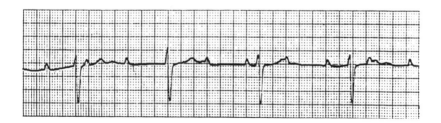

a. Perform cardioversion
b. Arrange for pacemaker placement
c. Give digoxin
d. Give propranolol
e. Give lidocaine

167. A 48-year-old male with a history of hypercholesterolemia presents to the ER after 1 h of substernal chest pain, nausea, and sweating. His ECG is shown below. There is no history of hypertension, stroke, or any other serious illness. Which of the following therapies is inappropriate?

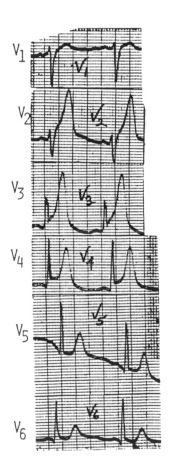

a. Aspirin
b. Beta blocker
c. Calcium channel blocker
d. Morphine
e. Nitroglycerin
f. Primary percutaneous coronary intervention

168. A 55-year-old obese woman develops pressure-like substernal chest pain lasting 1 h. Quickly obtained additional history includes the fact that she works as a housekeeper, which requires a considerable amount of lifting and exertion. Recently she had a somewhat similar pain at night after lying down. There is a positive family history of gallstones (mother and sister). Her ECG is shown below. Which of the following is the most likely diagnosis?

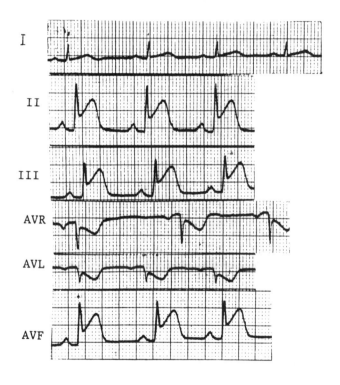

a. Costochondritis
b. Acute anterior myocardial infarction
c. Acute inferior myocardial infarction
d. Pericarditis
e. Gastroesophageal reflux
f. Cholecystitis

169. A 50-year-old construction worker continues to have an elevated blood pressure of 160/95 even after a third agent is added to his antihypertensive regimen. Physical exam is normal, electrolytes are normal, and the patient is taking no over-the-counter medications. Which of the following is the next helpful step for this patient?

a. Check pill count
b. Evaluate for Cushing syndrome
c. Check chest x-ray for coarctation of the aorta
d. Obtain a renal angiogram
e. Obtain an adrenal CT scan

170. A 35-year-old male complains of substernal chest pain aggravated by inspiration and relieved by sitting up. He has a history of tuberculosis. Lung fields are clear to auscultation, and heart sounds are somewhat distant. Chest x-ray shows an enlarged cardiac silhouette. Which of the following is the best next step in evaluation?

a. Right lateral decubitus film
b. Cardiac catheterization
c. Echocardiogram
d. Serial ECGs
e. Thallium stress test

171. A 42-year-old female suspected of having acute pericarditis has suddenly developed jugular venous distention and hypotension. The ECG shows electrical alternans. Which of the following is the most likely additional physical finding?

a. Basilar rales halfway up both posterior lung fields
b. S_3 gallop
c. Pulsus paradoxus
d. Strong apical beat

172. A 43-year-old woman with a 1-year history of episodic leg edema and dyspnea is noted to have clubbing of the fingers. Her ECG is shown below. Which of the following is the most likely diagnosis?

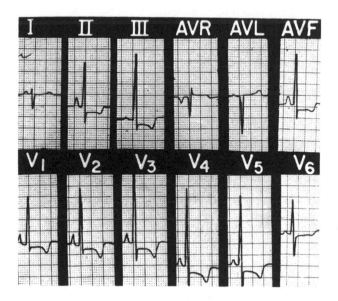

a. Inferior wall myocardial infarction
b. Right bundle branch block
c. Acute pericarditis
d. Wolff-Parkinson-White syndrome
e. Cor pulmonale

173. A 62-year-old male with underlying COPD develops a viral upper respiratory infection and begins taking an over-the-counter decongestant. Shortly thereafter he experiences palpitations and presents to the emergency room, where the following rhythm strip is obtained. The rhythm strip demonstrates which of the following?

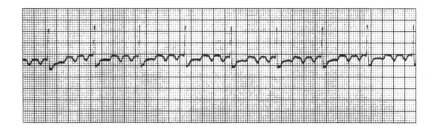

a. Normal sinus rhythm
b. Junctional rhythm
c. Atrial flutter with 4:1 atrioventricular block
d. Paroxysmal atrial tachycardia with 2:1 atrioventricular block
e. Complete heart block with 2:1 atrioventricular block

174. An asymptomatic 30-year-old female postdoc was noted by her gynecologist to have a cardiac murmur. She was referred for an echocardiogram, with results reported to her as showing mitral valve prolapse. The patient desires more information and now comes to you. Which of the following is true about her condition?

a. Displacement of one or both mitral valve leaflets posteriorly into the left atrium occurs during systole
b. Migration of the systolic click and systolic murmur toward the first heart sound will occur during squatting
c. Prophylactic beta blocker therapy is indicated
d. Significant mitral regurgitation is likely to occur (>50% chance) sometime in her life
e. Restriction of vigorous exercise is advised to reduce the risk of sudden cardiac death

175. You are reviewing a number of patients with congenital heart disease with specific attention to whether or not they need antibiotic prophylaxis for dental work. Who does not require endocarditis prophylaxis (i.e., which condition is at low risk for development of infective endocarditis)?

a. Coarctation of the aorta
b. Ventricular septal defect
c. Atrial septal defect
d. Patent ductus arteriosus
e. Hypertrophic cardiomyopathy
f. Prosthetic heart valve

176. An 80-year-old with a past history of myocardial infarction is found to have left bundle branch block on ECG. She is asymptomatic, with blood pressure 130/80, lungs clear to auscultation, and no leg edema. On cardiac auscultation, which of the following is the most likely finding?

a. Fixed (wide) split S_2
b. Paradoxical (reversed) split S_2
c. S_3
d. S_4
e. Opening snap
f. Midsystolic click

177. An ECG is brought to you with notation of this being a 62-year-old male with small cell carcinoma of the lung and hyponatremia. The electrocardiographic finding most likely to occur in this case is which of the following?

a. No abnormal change
b. Shortened PR interval
c. Prolonged PR interval
d. Convex elevation of the J point (Osborn wave)
e. Diffuse ST-segment elevation

DIRECTIONS: Each group of questions below consists of lettered options followed by a set of numbered items. For each numbered item, select the **one** lettered option with which it is **most** closely associated. Each lettered option may be used once, more than once, or not at all.

Questions 178–180

You are working in the university student health clinic, seeing adolescents and young adults for urgent care problems, but you remain attuned to the possibility of more serious underlying disease. For each of the numbered cases below, select the associated valvular or related heart disease.

a. Tricuspid stenosis
b. Tricuspid regurgitation
c. Mitral stenosis
d. Mitral regurgitation
e. Aortic regurgitation (insufficiency)
f. Aortic stenosis
g. Hypertrophic cardiomyopathy
h. Pulmonic stenosis
i. Pulmonic regurgitation (insufficiency)

178. This tall, thin 19-year-old white female with little previous health care complains primarily of decreased vision. You note a strong pulse, blood pressure of 180/70, and a high-pitched, blowing, diastolic decrescendo murmur.

179. A 23-year-old graduate student comes in with extreme fatigue and a vague sense of ill feeling over the past few weeks. He states that he has been under much stress recently, and in fact is slightly agitated. On exam, BP is 110/70, pulse is 100, and temperature is 100.5°F (38.0°C). The neck veins are distended with prominent v waves. A holosystolic murmur is heard at the left sternal border, which intensifies on inspiration.

180. An 18-year-old male is sent over from his physical education class due to his symptoms of dizziness and palpitations after exercise. The instructor thinks he may be faking this to get out of future activities. Vital signs are within normal limits. A rapidly rising carotid pulse is noted. On auscultation an S_4 is heard along with a harsh systolic crescendo-decrescendo murmur, beginning well after S_1, best noted at the lower left sternal border.

Questions 181–183

While on call in the hospital, you become involved in the following emergent situations. For each of the numbered cases below, choose the best next step in antiarrhythmic management from the following choices.

a. Amiodarone
b. Atropine
c. Digoxin
d. Diltiazem
e. Isoproterenol
f. Lidocaine
g. Metoprolol
h. Observation
i. Quinidine

181. A 72-year-old male presents with a 2-h history of chest pain; acute ST segment elevation in leads II, III, and a VF; and sinus bradycardia at a rate of 40, with hypotension.

182. A 58-year-old female smoker was admitted to the ICU with respiratory distress due to pneumonia. This was complicated by an anterior myocardial infarction, with management including cautious use of beta blockers. She now develops 10 to 12 PVCs per hour, occasional couplets, and a few short runs of ventricular tachycardia, although blood pressure and oxygen saturation remain stable.

183. A 60-year-old male during his first day post–myocardial infarction in the CCU develops an accelerated idioventricular rhythm, with rate of 80.

Questions 184–186

In the outpatient setting, you are treating a number of patients with hypertension. Knowing the adverse possibilities along with the benefits of each antihypertensive can help you achieve compliance and therefore blood pressure control. For each of the numbered cases below, select the most significant listed adverse effect of the antihypertensive and/or cardiac agent in question.

a. Increased triglyceride levels
b. Peripheral edema
c. Lupus-like syndrome
d. Cough
e. Gynecomastia
f. Rebound hypertension
g. First-dose syncope
h. Urinary retention

184. A 45-year-old white female has been on a diuretic, but BP remains elevated at 145/95, leading to the proposed addition of lisinopril. This key potential adverse effect should be discussed.

185. A 58-year-old African American male long-haul truck driver has significant hypertension, still not controlled on a diuretic plus calcium channel blocker. Clonidine is being considered as the next medication, but in this patient the concerns are sedation, sexual dysfunction, and this side effect.

186. A 68-year-old male with advanced CHF and BP 142/92 will have spironolactone added to his regimen, but should be informed about this possible side effect.

Questions 187–189

You have been assigned to review the ECGs for the group this month. The only background information available to you is as given on each ECG. For each of the numbered cases (ECGs) below, select the electrocardiographic finding, from among those listed, which is most likely to occur.

a. Electrical alternans
b. Widened QRS complex
c. ST segment scooping
d. Shortened QT interval
e. Prolonged QT interval
f. Prominent U waves

187. A 64-year-old female, diagnosed with venous insufficiency, is on furosemide.

188. A 70-year-old male, diagnosed with mild chronic renal insufficiency plus CHF, is on metoprolol, losartan, and spironolactone; he's allergic to furosemide.

189. A 52-year-old otherwise healthy female is postop subtotal thyroidectomy for persistent toxic multinodular goiter.

Cardiology

Answers

143. The answer is b. *(Kasper, pp 1444–1447.)* This patient presents with unstable angina, a change from the previous chronic stable state in that chest pain has become more frequent and more severe. Antithrombotic therapy with intravenous heparin is indicated, along with additional antiplatelet therapy using clopidogrel. Subcutaneous administration of low-molecular-weight heparin (such as enoxaparin) is an alternative. There is no role for digoxin, as this may increase myocardial oxygen consumption and exacerbate the situation. Thrombolytic therapy is reserved for the treatment, typically within 6 h, of ECG-documented myocardial infarction and does not reduce cardiac events in the setting of unstable angina. A more aggressive approach is early interventional cardiac catheterization with angioplasty and/or stent placement, possibly in conjunction with glycoprotein IIb/IIIa inhibitors.

144. The answer is a. *(Kasper, pp 1332–1333.)* The right coronary artery provides the circulation to most of the inferior myocardium. At its proximal end in 60% of patients it supplies the sinoatrial node via the SA artery, and toward its distal end in 90% of patients it supplies the AV node via the posterior descending coronary artery. Thus, occlusion of the right coronary artery can cause ischemia of the AV node in particular and possibly the SA node, with AV block and/or bradycardia, as well as symptoms of an inferior MI, as seen in this patient. AV block can occur with anterior MI related to LAD occlusion, but this generally implies a greater area of myocardial involvement and hemodynamic instability.

145. The answer is b. *(Kasper, pp 1449–1450.)* The classic presentation of acute myocardial infarction (MI) involves heavy or crushing substernal chest pain or pressure. However, 15 to 20% of infarctions may be painless, with the greatest incidence in diabetics and the elderly. Dyspnea or weakness may initially predominate in these patients. Other presentations include altered mental status, the appearance of an arrhythmia, or hypotension. Diabetics are likely to have abnormal or absent pain response to myocardial ischemia due to generalized autonomic nervous system dys-

CardiologyAnswers105

function. The other choices have no specific link to greater likelihood of a silent MI.

146. The answer is d. (*Kasper, p 1448.*) This case describes Prinzmetal's variant angina, a syndrome of ischemic pain that classically occurs at rest rather than with exertion and is associated with transient ST-segment elevation due to focal coronary artery spasm (most commonly involving the right coronary, although in this example, with precordial lead findings, the left anterior descending is more likely). The pain is usually not preceded by a period of chronic stable angina. Exercise stress testing is unlikely to be diagnostic in Prinzmetal's, and results may be difficult to interpret in young females in general. Coronary angiography demonstrating transient coronary artery spasm is the diagnostic hallmark of this condition. Nitrates and calcium channel blockers are the mainstays of treatment. Regarding the other listed choices, echocardiography and anti-inflammatory therapy allude to the diagnosis of pericarditis; however, in this condition ST-segment elevation should occur diffusely, and the pain is not relieved by nitroglycerin. EGD and proton pump inhibitor therapy allude to the diagnosis of gastroesophageal reflux, which may produce pain upon lying down, but should not yield ECG changes; nitroglycerin conceivably could relieve the pain of associated esophageal spasm. There is nothing specific here to warrant the chest CT or IV heparin treatment of pulmonary embolism.

147. The answer is c. (*Kasper, pp 1417–1418.*) The history and physical exam are consistent with post–cardiac injury syndrome (in the past also known as Dressler syndrome, or postmyocardial infarction syndrome). This generally benign, self-limited syndrome comprises an autoimmune pleuritis, pneumonitis, or pericarditis characterized by fever and pleuritic chest pain, with onset days to 6 weeks post–cardiac injury with blood in the pericardial cavity, as after a cardiac operation, cardiac trauma, or MI. Therefore the most effective therapy is a nonsteroidal anti-inflammatory drug or occasionally a glucocorticoid. Infection such as bacterial pneumonia, which would require antibiotics, would typically cause dyspnea, cough with sputum production, and rales on lung auscultation. Pulmonary embolus, which would require anticoagulation, would cause dyspnea and tachypnea, often in conjunction with physical findings of heat, swelling, and pain in the leg consistent with deep vein thrombosis. Angina or recurrent myocardial infarction is always a concern post-MI (and what the patient usually fears in this situation), but the nature of the pain—here pleuritic rather than pressure-like—and the unchanged ECG are fairly reassuring and mitigate against an increase in antianginal therapy. Anxiety can be present but would not cause fever.

148. The answer is d. *(Kasper, pp 1370–1371.)* Use of the Framingham criteria (eight major and seven minor) is one method by which to organize the signs and symptoms for the diagnosis of congestive heart failure. Major criteria include paroxysmal nocturnal dyspnea, neck vein distension, rales, cardiomegaly, acute pulmonary edema, S_3 gallop, increased venous pressure, and positive hepatojugular reflux. Minor criteria include extremity edema, night cough, dyspnea on exertion, hepatomegaly, pleural effusion, vital capacity reduced by one-third from normal, and tachycardia of 120 or more beats per minute. In addition, weight loss of 4.5 kg or more over 5 days of treatment may be considered as a major or minor criterion. To establish a clinical diagnosis of CHF by this method, at least one major and two minor criteria are required.

149. The answer is a. *(Kasper, pp 1372–1375.)* Angiotensin-converting enzyme inhibitors have been shown to prevent or retard the development of heart failure in patients with left ventricular dysfunction and to reduce long-term mortality when begun shortly after an MI, via inhibition of the renin-angiotensin system and reduction of preload and afterload. Thus they play a central role in heart failure management. An angiotensin II receptor blocker may be substituted. Beta blockers are typically the next addition, also with evidence supporting reduction in rehospitalization for CHF and future cardiac events. Loop or thiazide diuretics are administered to those with fluid accumulation. The aldosterone antagonist spironolactone is indicated in more advanced CHF. Digoxin is reserved for those with clear-cut systolic dysfunction, especially with atrial flutter or fibrillation with rapid ventricular response. The nitrate-hydralazine combination is also an option in ACE inhibitor–intolerant patients, almost always in advanced cases. Calcium channel blockers are not indicated for heart failure or routinely post-MI. General therapeutic measures include salt restriction and regular moderate exercise. Patient preferences are important to consider but should not keep you from giving your best medical recommendation, which the patient can then decide to accept or not.

150. The answer is b. (*Kasper, pp 34, 1410.*) Peripartum (or postpartum) cardiomyopathy may occur during the last trimester of pregnancy or within 6 months of delivery, but most commonly in the month before or after delivery. The most common demographics are multiparity, African American race, and age greater than 30. About half of patients will recover completely, with most of the rest improving, although the mortality rate is quoted as 10 to 20%. Current advice is to avoid future pregnancies due to the risk of recurrence. Treatment is as for other dilated cardiomyopathies, except that ACE inhibitors are contraindicated in pregnancy.

151. The answer is d. (*Kasper, pp 1325, 1436–1437.*) Left ventricular hypertrophy and, in particular, preexisting ST-segment depression greater than 1 mm from any cause (such as with bundle branch block, a paced rhythm, or WPW) are contraindications to routine stress testing. New ST-segment depression is the most common stress test–induced evidence of myocardial ischemia and would be difficult to assess if the ST segment is already abnormal. Nuclear imaging would be indicated instead. Anxiety, mildly elevated blood pressure, or suspected angina would not preclude a stress test. Cardiac auscultation in this case suggests just an innocent flow murmur. Pathologic murmurs, however, warrant caution. Aortic stenosis, in particular, would be a contraindication to stress testing. This would manifest as a harsh systolic crescendo-decrescendo murmur, usually heard best at the upper right sternal border with radiation to the carotids.

152. The answer is a. (*Kasper, p 1397.*) The classic triad of symptoms of aortic stenosis are exertional dyspnea, angina pectoris, and syncope. Physical findings include a narrow pulse pressure and systolic murmur as described in answer a (rather than the aortic insufficiency murmur of answer b, the mitral regurgitation murmur of answer c, or the mitral valve prolapse click of answer d).

153. The answer is a. (*Kasper, pp 1390–1391.*) The history and physical exam findings are consistent with mitral stenosis. Dyspnea may be present secondary to pulmonary edema; palpitations are often related to atrial arrhythmias (PACs, PAT, atrial flutter, or fibrillation); hemoptysis may occur as a consequence of pulmonary hypertension with rupture of bronchial veins. A diastolic rumbling apical murmur is characteristic. An accentuated first heart sound and opening snap may also be present. The etiology of mitral stenosis is usually rheumatic, rarely congenital. Two-thirds of patients afflicted are women.

154. The answer is c. *(Kasper, pp 1308–1311, 1385–1386, 1397–1400.)* A holosystolic murmur at the mid-left sternal border is the murmur most characteristic of a ventricular septal defect. Both the murmur of ventricular septal defect and the murmur of mitral regurgitation are enhanced by exercise and diminished by amyl nitrite. Answers a, b, d, and e describe the usual findings in aortic stenosis, atrial septal defect, aortic insufficiency, and patent ductus arteriosus, respectively.

155. The answer is e. *(Kasper, p 1343.)* PVCs are common in patients with and without heart disease, and they are detected in 60% of adult males on Holter monitoring. Occasional unifocal PVCs do not specifically suggest any of the underlying diseases described.

156. The answer is e. *(Kasper, pp 1343–1344.)* Minimally symptomatic PVCs do not require treatment. Antiarrhythmic therapy in this setting has not been shown to reduce sudden cardiac death or overall mortality. A beta blocker would be the best choice if symptoms began to interfere with daily activities.

157. The answer is e. *(Kasper, pp 1345–1346, 2376–2377.)* Aspirin or other antiplatelet therapy alone might be sufficient for a stroke patient without the complicating factor of atrial fibrillation. However, in patients with atrial fibrillation and a risk factor (including previous stroke or TIAs, hypertension, LV dysfunction/CHF, coronary artery disease, rheumatic mitral valvular disease, prosthethic valve, diabetes, or thyrotoxicosis), the incidence of stroke averages 5% per year (up to 15% per year in those with multiple risk factors); therapeutic anticoagulation with warfarin (Coumadin) reduces this risk to a greater extent than the use of antiplatelet agents (warfarin 68% compared to aspirin 21%). The target INR is generally 2.0 to 3.0, but more specifically 2.5 to 3.0 in those over age 75, and 2.5 to 3.5 with prosthetic valves. Depending on left atrial diameter (i.e., if <4.5 cm on echocardiogram), this particular patient might be a candidate for medical or electrical cardioversion, which requires pretreatment with Coumadin for 3 weeks (if the atrial fibrillation has been present for over 48 h or is of unknown onset). Alternatively, a transesophageal echocardiogram

(TEE) could be performed to exclude the presence of left atrial thrombus, followed by cardioversion and then maintenance warfarin anticoagulation.

158. The answer is c. (*Kasper, pp 1345, 1347, 1351.*) Paroxysmal supraventricular tachycardia due to AV nodal reentry typically displays a narrow QRS complex without clearly discernible P waves, with a rate in the 160 to 190 range. The atrial rate is faster in atrial flutter, typically with a classic sawtooth pattern of P waves, with AV conduction ratios most commonly 2:1 or 4:1, leading to ventricular rates of 150 or 75 per min. Atrial fibrillation would show an irregularly irregular rhythm without discrete P waves. Wide QRS complexes with rate greater than 100 would be expected in ventricular tachycardia.

159. The answer is c. (*Kasper, pp 1482–1483.*) Abdominal aortic aneurysms occur in 1 to 2% of men older than 50 years and to a lesser extent in women. They are commonly asymptomatic, and acute rupture may occur without warning. Alternatively, they may expand and become painful, with pain as a harbinger of rupture. The risk of rupture increases with the size of the aneurysm, with the 5-year risk reported as 1 to 2% if less than 5 cm, but 20 to 40% if greater than 5 cm. Other studies indicate that in patients with AAAs less than 5.5 cm, there is no difference in long-term mortality rate between those followed with ultrasound and those who undergo elective aneurysmal repair. Therefore, operative repair is typically recommended in asymptomatic individuals if the AAA diameter is greater than 5.5 cm; other indications for surgery are rapid expansion or onset of symptoms. With careful preoperative evaluation and postoperative care the surgical mortality rate should be less than 1 to 2%. Endovascular stent grafts for infrarenal AAAs are achieving success in selected patients.

160. The answer is g. (*Kasper, pp 1337–1338.*) This ECG shows Mobitz type I second-degree AV block, also known as Wenckebach phenomenon, characterized by progressive PR interval prolongation prior to block of an atrial impulse. This rhythm generally does not require therapy. It may be seen in normal individuals; other causes include inferior MI and drug intoxications such as from digoxin, beta blockers, or calcium channel blockers. Even in the post-MI setting, it is usually stable, although it has the potential to progress to higher-degree AV block with consequent need for pacemaker.

161. The answer is d. *(Kasper, pp 1622–1623.)* The standard approach to ventricular fibrillation or hypotensive ventricular tachycardia involves defibrillation with 200 joules, then 300, then 360, followed if needed by epinephrine 1 mg IV push every 3 to 5 min. If persistent, such ventricular arrhythmias lead to consideration of amiodarone 150 mg IV push or lidocaine 1.0 to 1.5 mg/kg IV push. In addition, magnesium sulfate 1 to 2 g IV may be given in torsade de pointes or when arrhythmia due to hypomagnesemia is suspected. Procainamide up to 30 mg/min (maximum total 17 mg/kg) is given to patients with intermittent return of a pulse or non-VF rhythm, but then recurrence of VF/VT. A precordial thump may be considered at the outset in this case, but there is insufficient evidence to recommend its use or avoidance.

162. The answer is d. *(Kasper, pp 1483–1484.)* This case description is classic for aortic dissection, other than the fact that it is more common in men than women. Aortic insufficiency is common with proximal dissection, as is hypertension and evidence of CHF. Hypotension may be present in severe cases. More distal dissection can lead to obstruction of other major arteries with neurological symptoms (carotids), bowel ischemia, or renal compromise. With this diagnosis, the first line of defense in emergent therapy is parenteral beta blocker therapy, such as with metoprolol, propranolol, esmolol, or labetalol, while seeking more diagnostic details with echocardiography and/or CT scan (or possibly MRI). After beta blockade is established, nitroprusside is commonly used to titrate systolic blood pressure to less than 120. Urgent surgery is then usually needed. The other answers involve therapy for diagnoses of CHF, which is present but not the primary concern; angina/MI, which is less likely; subacute bacterial endocarditis; and acute pulmonary embolism, for which there is little evidence.

163. The answer is b. *(Kasper, pp 1478, 1480.)* This patient manifests malignant hypertension with diastolic blood pressure greater than 130 and acute (or ongoing) target organ damage. She shows one subset of such damage, namely, hypertensive encephalopathy, including headache, visual disturbance, and altered mental status. Immediate therapy with nitroprusside is indicated in the ICU setting, although it would be avoided if renal insufficiency were present. Other options include intravenous nitroglycerin, fenoldopam, or enalaprilat. Intravenous labetalol is often used in hypertensive urgencies, but, as a beta blocker, it is relatively contraindicated in asthma. An oral medication such as clonidine would be slow-acting and difficult to administer in a lethargic patient. Sublingual nifedipine is no longer advised due to increased potential for overshoot hypotension with adverse cardiovascular events such as MI or stroke and ischemic optic neuropathy.

164. The answer is b. (*Kasper, pp 1977–1979.*) This 18-year-old presents with classic features of rheumatic fever. (See reference for updated Jones criteria.) His clinical manifestations include arthritis, fever, and murmur (here aortic insufficiency, although mitral regurgitation is more common). A subcutaneous nodule is noted, and a rash of erythema marginatum is described. These subcutaneous nodules are pea-sized and usually seen over extensor tendons. The rash is usually pink with clear centers and serpiginous margins. Laboratory data includes an elevated erythrocyte sedimentation rate as usually occurs in rheumatic fever. The ECG shows evidence of first-degree AV block. An antistreptolysin O antibody is necessary to diagnose the disease by documenting prior streptococcal infection.

165. The answer is a. (*Kasper, pp 1347–1349.*) Vagotonic manuevers such as carotid massage or the Valsalva manuever could certainly be tried first. If these are unsuccessful, adenosine, with its excellent safety profile and extremely short half-life, is the drug of choice for supraventricular tachycardia, at an initial dose of 6 mg. Dosage can be repeated if necessary a few minutes later at 12 mg. Verapamil is the next alternative; if the initial dose of 2.5 to 5 mg does not yield conversion, one or two additional boluses 10 min apart can be used. Diltiazem and digoxin may be useful in rate control and conversion, but have a much slower onset of action. Electrical cardioversion would be reserved for hemodynamically unstable patients. Lidocaine is useful in ventricular, but not in supraventricular, arrhythmias.

166. The answer is b. (*Kasper, pp 1336–1341.*) The ECG shows complete heart block. Although at first glance the P waves and QRS complexes may appear related, on closer inspection they are completely independent of each other (i.e., dissociated). Complete heart block in the setting of acute myocardial infarction requires at least temporary, and often permanent, transvenous pacemaker placement. Atropine may be used as a temporary measure. You would certainly want to avoid digoxin, beta blockers, or any other medication that promotes bradycardia. There is no indication on this strip for cardioversion such as for atrial fibrillation/flutter or ventricular tachycardia/fibrillation. Lidocaine would be relatively contraindicated in that it might suppress the ventricular pacemaker, leading to asystole.

167. The answer is c. *(Kasper, pp 1452–1454.)* The ECG shows acute ST-segment elevations in the anterior precordial leads. The symptoms have persisted for only 1 h, so the patient is a candidate for primary percutaneous coronary intervention (angioplasty and/or stenting) or thrombolytic therapy, depending on the setting. Aspirin should be given. Nitroglycerin and morphine are indicated for pain control. Beta blockers reduce pain, limit infarct size, and decrease ventricular arrhythmias. There is no role for calcium channel blockers in this acute setting; in fact, short-acting dihydropyridines may increase mortality.

168. The answer is c. *(Kasper, pp 1316–1318.)* The ECG shows ST-segment elevation in inferior leads II, III, and a VF with reciprocal ST depression in aVL, which is highly consistent with an acute inferior MI. An anterior MI would produce ST-segment elevation in the precordial leads. Pericarditis classically produces pleuritic chest pain and diffuse ST segment elevation (except aVR) on ECG. Costochondritis, gastroesophageal reflux, and cholecystitis are confounding considerations raised by the history and can all cause the symptom of substernal chest pain, but not these ECG findings.

169. The answer is a. *(Kasper, p 1479.)* The most common cause of refractory hypertension is nonadherence to the medication regimen. A history from the patient is useful, and pill count is the best compliance check. Cushing's disease, coarctation of the aorta, renal artery stenosis, and primary aldosteronism are secondary causes that could result in refractory hypertension, but no clues to these diagnoses are apparent on physical exam or lab.

170. The answer is c. *(Kasper, pp 1414–1415.)* The patient's pleuritic chest pain that is relieved by sitting up is most likely due to pericarditis. A pericardial friction rub may initially be present, then disappear, with the heart sounds becoming fainter as an effusion develops. Lung sounds are typically clear. An enlarged cardiac silhouette without other chest x-ray findings of heart failure suggests pericardial effusion.

Echocardiography is the most sensitive, specific way of determining whether pericardial fluid is present. The effusion appears as an echo-free space between the moving epicardium and stationary pericardium. It is unnecessary to perform cardiac catheterization for the purpose of evaluating pericardial effusion. Radionuclide scanning is not a preferred method for demonstrating pericardial fluid.

171. The answer is c. (*Kasper, pp 1367–1368.*) The patient has developed cardiac tamponade, a condition in which pericardial fluid under increased pressure impedes diastolic filling, resulting in reduced cardiac output and hypotension. On exam there is elevation of jugular venous pressure. The jugular venous pulse shows a sharp x descent, the inward impulse seen at the time of the carotid pulsation. An important confirmatory clue to cardiac tamponade on exam is pulsus paradoxus, a greater than normal (10 mmHg) inspiratory decline in systolic arterial pressure. In contrast to pulmonary edema, the lungs are usually clear. Neither a strong apical beat nor an S_3 gallop would be expected in tamponade.

172. The answer is e. (*Kasper, pp 1314, 1377–1378, 1404–1405.*) Cor pulmonale indicates a pulmonary abnormality, leading to pulmonary hypertension, with right ventricular enlargement and consequent right ventricular dysfunction. Its causes include diseases leading to hypoxic vasoconstriction, as in cystic fibrosis; occlusion of the pulmonary vasculature, as in pulmonary thromboembolism; other pulmonary vascular problems, such as the collagen-vascular disease vasculitides; parenchymal destruction, as in sarcoidosis; COPD; and primary pulmonary hypertension. With a chronic increase in afterload, the RV hypertrophies, dilates, and fails. The electrocardiographic findings, as illustrated in the question, include tall, peaked P waves in leads II, III, and aVF, which indicate right atrial enlargement; tall R waves in leads V_1 to V_3 and a deep S wave in V_6 with associated ST-T wave changes, which indicate right ventricular hypertrophy; and right axis deviation. Right bundle branch block occurs in 15% of patients.

173. The answer is c. (*Kasper, p 1347.*) The rhythm strip in the question reveals atrial flutter with 4:1 atrioventricular (AV) block. Atrial flutter is characterized by an atrial rate of 250 to 350/min; the electrocardiogram typically reveals a sawtooth baseline configuration due to the flutter waves.

In the strip, every fourth atrial depolarization is conducted through the AV node, resulting in a ventricular rate of 75/min (although 2:1 conduction is more commonly seen).

174. The answer is a. *(Kasper, pp 1395–1396.)* The fundamental defect in mitral valve prolapse is an abnormality of the valve's connective tissue with secondary proliferation of myxomatous tissue. The redundant leaflet(s) prolapses toward the left atrium in systole, which results in the auscultated click and murmur and characteristic echocardiographic findings. Any maneuver that reduces left ventricular size, such as standing or the Valsalva maneuver, allows the click and murmur to occur earlier in systole; conversely, conditions that increase left ventricular size, such as squatting or propranolol administration, delay the onset of the click and murmur. Severe mitral regurgitation is an uncommon complication. Most patients with MVP have a benign prognosis, and, in the absence of mitral regurgitation or arrhythmias, reassurance is the key point in management. Antibiotic prophylaxis to prevent endocarditis is reserved for those with the systolic murmur of mitral regurgitation and/or thickening of mitral valve leaflets on echocardiography. Beta blocker therapy is reserved for symptoms, including those related to arrhythmias.

175. The answer is c. *(Kasper, pp 739–740.)* In general, congenital heart disease patients are at higher risk of infective endocarditis, except for isolated secundum atrial septal defect and the following if surgically corrected: ASD, VSD, PDA, and pulmonic stenosis. High-risk conditions include prosthetic heart valves, coarctation of the aorta, patent ductus arteriosus, and Marfan's syndrome. Moderate risk is conferred by ventricular septal defect, congenital or acquired valvular disease (including mitral valve prolapse with regurgitation and/or thickened leaflets), and hypertrophic cardiomyopathy. Low risk is seen in ASD, post-CABG, with pacemakers or AICDs, and in MVP without regurgitation.

176. The answer is b. *(Kasper, pp 1307–1308.)* Normally, the second heart sound (S_2) is composed of aortic closure followed by pulmonic closure. Because inspiration increases blood return to the right side of the heart, pulmonic closure is delayed, which results in normal splitting of S_2 during inspiration. Paradoxical splitting of S_2, however, refers to splitting of S_2 that is narrowed instead of widened with inspiration consequent to a delayed aortic closure. Paradoxical splitting can result from any electrical or mechanical event that delays left ventricular systole. Thus, aortic stenosis and hypertension, which increase resistance to systolic ejection of blood, delay closure of the aortic valve. Acute ischemia from angina or acute myocardial infarction also can delay ejection of blood from the left ventricle. The most common cause of paradoxical splitting—left bundle branch block—delays electrical activation of the left ventricle. Right bundle branch block results in a wide splitting of S_2 that widens further during inspiration. An S_3 is typically heard with congestive heart failure, an S_4 with hypertension, an opening snap with mitral stenosis, and a midsystolic click with mitral valve prolapse.

177. The answer is a. *(Kasper, p 1319.)* At serum sodium levels compatible with life, neither hyponatremia nor hypernatremia result in any characteristic ECG changes, although nonspecific ST-T changes could occur. A convex elevation of the J point (Osborn wave) is seen in hypothermia.

178–180. The answers are 178-e, 179-b, 180-g. *(Kasper, pp 1399–1400, 2329–2330, 1402, 1410–1411.)* The person *in the first of these three cases* displays the classic triad of features of Marfan's syndrome: (1) long, thin extremities, possibly with arachnodactyly or other skeletal changes; (2) reduced vision as a result of lens dislocations; and (3) aortic root dilatation or aneurysm. The diastolic murmur described is characteristic of aortic regurgitation (insufficiency), accompanied by the peripheral signs of water-hammer pulse and widened pulse pressure. *In the second of these three cases*, the neck vein and cardiac exam findings are consistent with tricuspid regurgitation. Recall that inspiration increases right heart volume and therefore augments the auscultated murmur. The symptoms and low-grade fever raise the suspicion of its cause being infective endocarditis. Further history and physical signs of IV drug abuse should be sought. TR may proceed to right heart failure. *The final case* describes a patient with hypertrophic cardiomyopathy. Dyspnea is also a common complaint. The worst-case scenario is sudden cardiac death as the first manifestation of the disease, often occurring with or after physical exertion. Diagnosis is confirmed by echocardiography, which shows diffuse left ventricular hypertrophy with preferential hypertrophy of the interventricular septum. The murmur may be more holosystolic and heard at the apex, making it difficult to distinguish from mitral regurgitation. Management includes avoidance of strenuous exertion, good hydration, and beta blockers. First-degree relatives should also be screened with echocardiography.

181–183. The answers are 181-b, 182-a, 183-h. *(Kasper, pp 1343–1344, 1351–1353, 1456–1457.)* The person *in the first of these three cases* displays sinus bradycardia, a common rhythm disturbance in acute inferior MI secondary to increased vagal tone. With associated hypotension, atropine should be given. Intravenous inotropic agents are generally not required. *In the second of these three cases,* cardiac ischemia, the level of ventricular ectopy, in particular the ventricular tachycardia (which is hemodynamically stable at this point and not requiring electrical cardioversion), warrants treatment with IV amiodarone. The approach to PVCs has changed in recent years, in part due to the realization that antiarrhythmics can potentially exacerbate rather than help the ectopy. Prophylactic antiarrhythmics such as lidocaine are no longer recommended. Infrequent, sporadic PVCs do not require treatment. No rigid criteria for mandatory treatment (e.g., >5 PVCs/min, multifocal origin, or early diastolic "R on T" occurrence) are currently in force. PVCs > 10/min and complexity such as couplets have been associated with increased mortality, but typically in association with LV dysfunction, such that the antiarrhythmic decision is based on assessing the cardiac status as a whole. Beta blockers are usually given post-MI and may provide some antiarrhythmic benefit. *The final case* points to the fact that accelerated idioventricular rhythm ("slow V tach") with rate 60 to 100 develops in 25% of post-MI patients. Enhanced automaticity of Purkinje fibers is considered the most likely etiology. This is usually considered a benign rhythm, unlikely to degenerate into ventricular tachycardia or other serious arrhythmia, so only observation and monitoring are necessary.

184–186. The answers are 184-d, 185-f, 186-e. *(Kasper, pp 1472–1478.)* Lisinopril and other angiotensin-converting enzyme inhibitors may cause angioedema, acute renal failure in the presence of renal artery stenosis, hyperkalemia, and other uncommon adverse effects. However, the most common and aggravating side effect is dry cough, occurring in 5 to 10% of patients. The centrally acting agent clonidine is noted for rebound hypertension upon discontinuing the drug, probably secondary to an increase in norepinephrine release. It would not be favored in the setting of an occupation or lifestyle predisposed to erratic adherence to the regimen. The aldosterone (mineralocorticoid) antagonist spironolactone may cause gynecomastia and impotence in men and irregular menses in females, along with hyperkalemia. The other listed adverse effects allude to beta blockers (increased triglyceride levels plus reduction in HDL); calcium channel blockers and potent vasodilators such as minoxidil (fluid retention/peripheral edema); the vasodilator hydralazine (at high doses, lupus-like syndrome); and alpha blockers such as terazosin or doxazosin (first-dose syncope in <1%; they may improve, not cause, urinary retention).

187–189. The answers are 187-f, 188-b, 189-e. (*Kasper, pp 1318–1319.*) The use of a loop diuretic such as furosemide without potassium replacement suggests the likelihood of hypokalemia, which prolongs ventricular repolarization, resulting in flattened T waves and/or prominent U waves; hypokalemia may also cause ectopic beats or arrhythmias. Chronic renal insufficiency and the use (e.g., for CHF) of potassium-sparing agents such as the aldosterone antagonist spironolactone and the angiotensin II receptor blocker losartan (or an ACE inhibitor) suggest hyperkalemia. The earliest ECG change is usually the appearance of tall, peaked T waves, followed by AV conduction disturbances, flattened P waves, and a widened QRS complex. Thyroid surgery calls to attention the possibility of hypoparathyroidism with hypocalcemia, which prolongs the QT interval. Other conditions that may cause QT prolongation are the use of Class IA or III antiarrhythmics, intracranial bleeds, and the congenital long QT syndrome. Conversely, a shortened QT interval may be caused by hypercalcemia or digitalis glycosides. The latter is the classic cause of ST scooping. Electrical alternans, a beat-to-beat alternation in one or more components of the ECG, suggests pericardial effusion, usually with cardiac tamponade.

Endocrinology and Metabolic Disease

Questions

DIRECTIONS: Each item below contains a question followed by suggested responses. Select the **one best** response to each question.

190. A 50-year-old obese female is taking oral hypoglycemic agents. While being treated for an upper respiratory infection, she develops lethargy and is brought to the emergency room. On physical exam, there is no focal neurologic finding or neck rigidity. Laboratory results are as follows:

Na^-: 134 meq/L
K^-: 4.0 meq/L
HCO_3: 25 meq/L
Glucose: 900 mg/dL
BUN: 84 mg/dL
Creatinine: 3.0 mg/dL
BP: 120/80 sitting, 105/65 lying down

Which of the following is the most likely cause of this patient's coma?

a. Diabetic ketoacidosis
b. Hyperosmolar coma
c. Inappropriate ADH
d. Bacterial meningitis

191. A 67-year-old male is brought to the office by his wife. He is brought to the room in a wheelchair although he is usually ambulatory. During the history you find that he responds slowly or not at all when asked questions. On physical exam he is afebrile but has signs of dehydration such as dry mucous membranes, decreased skin turgor, and positive orthostatic blood pressure change. A finger-stick glucose check is unreadable on the monitor and a stat metabolic panel result is as follows:

Na$^-$: 128 meq/L
K$^-$: 3.9 meq/L
HCO$_3$: 24 meq/L
Glucose: 860 mg/dL
BUN: 60 mg/dL
Creatinine: 1.2 mg/dL

You send him to the hospital for admission. Initial treatment should consist of which of the following?

a. Intravenous fluids
b. Hypertonic saline
c. KCL 30 meq/h
d. Intraveneous antibiotics

192. A 50-year-old female is 5 ft 7 in. tall and weighs 185 lb. There is a family history of diabetes mellitus. Fasting blood glucose is 130 mg/dL and 145 mg/dL on two occasions. She is asymptomatic, and physical exam shows no abnormalities. Which of the following is the treatment of choice?

a. Observation
b. Medical nutrition therapy
c. Insulin
d. Oral hypoglycemic agent

193. A 30-year-old female complains of palpitations, fatigue, and insomnia. On physical exam, her extremities are warm and she is tachycardic. There is diffuse thyroid gland enlargement and proptosis. There is a thickening of the skin in the pretibial area (see photo). Which of the following lab values would you expect in this patient?

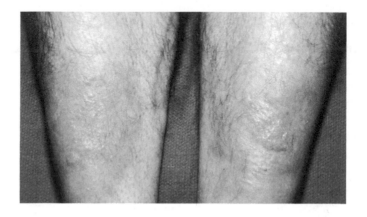

a. Increased TSH, total thyroxine, total T_3
b. Decreased TSH, increased total thyroxine
c. Increased T_3 uptake, decreased T_3
d. Decreased TSH, normal T_4

194. A 24-year-old female presents with complaints of anxiety, diarrhea, and heat intolerance. She has lost 20 lb in the past 3 months without really trying. Physical exam reveals a thin, anxious, white female in no distress, with mild proptosis and thyroid gland with diffuse enlargement. Thyroid function testing reveals:

TSH <0.03
Elevated T_4
Increased T_3 uptake

The most common diagnosis for this young woman's hyperthyroidism is which of the following?

a. Autoimmune disease
b. Benign tumor
c. Malignancy
d. Viral infection of the thyroid

195. You recently evaluated a 28-year-old G0 who presented with complaints of shakiness and heat intolerance. The patient plans to have children and is currently using no contraception. On exam you noted tachycardia with a HR of 102 and a fine tremor and proptosis. You now have the laboratory results and note a TSH <0.001, elevated total T_4 of 17.8, and increased T_3 uptake. The diagnosis of Graves' disease is made, and you consider treatment options. The treatment of choice in this patient, for whom remission from Graves' disease is possible, is which of the following?

a. Propylthiouracil
b. Radioactive iodine
c. Thyroid surgery
d. Oral corticosteroids

196. A 50-year-old female is evaluated for hypertension. Her blood pressure is 130/98. She complains of polyuria and of mild muscle weakness. She is on no diuretics or other blood pressure medication. On physical exam, the PMI is displaced to the sixth intercostal space. There is no sign of congestive heart failure and no edema. Laboratory values are as follows:

Na^-: 147 meq/dL
K^-: 2.3 meq/dL
Cl^-: 112 meq/dL
HCO_3: 27 meq/dL

The patient is on no other medication. She does not eat licorice. Which of the following will aid in diagnosis?

a. 24-h urine for cortisol
b. Urinary metanephrine
c. Plasma renin and aldosterone
d. Renal angiogram

197. A 36-year-old female presents with acute complaints of inability to lose weight despite low-calorie diet and daily exercise. She has also noticed that she is cold-intolerant. You note that she is wearing a jacket even though it is summer. She also reports constipation and hair loss. These symptoms have been worsening over the past 2 to 3 months. An elevated TSH and low total and free T_4 confirms your suspicion of hypothyroidism. You suspect the etiology of this patient's hypothyroidism is autoimmune thyroiditis. The diagnosis of autoimmune thyroiditis can be confirmed by which of the following?

a. Thyroid peroxidase antibody (TPO)
b. Antinuclear antibody
c. Thyroid uptake resin
d. Thyroid aspiration

198. On routine physical exam, a young woman is found to have a thyroid nodule. There is no pain, hoarseness, hemoptysis, or local symptoms. Serum TSH is normal. Which of the following is the best next step in evaluation?

a. Ultrasonography
b. Thyroid scan
c. Surgical resection
d. Fine needle aspiration of thyroid

199. A 55-year-old type 2 diabetic patient has lost weight and has had good control of his blood sugar on oral agents. He has a history of mild hypertension and hyperlipidemia. He asks for advice about an exercise program. Which of the following statements is correct?

a. Exercise should be avoided because it may cause foot trauma
b. An active lifestyle cannot slow the complications of diabetes
c. Vigorous exercise cannot precipitate hypoglycemia
d. A stress test should be recommended prior to beginning an exercise program

200. A newly diagnosed type 2 diabetic patient asks for clarification about dietary management. Which of the following is the best advice for this patient?

a. Restrict carbohydrates and eat a high-protein diet
b. Avoid sucrose altogether
c. Less than 10% of caloric intake should be saturated fat
d. Caloric intake should be very consistent from one day to another

201. As part of a review of systems, a 55-year-old male describes an inability to achieve erection. The patient has mild diabetes and is on a beta blocker for hypertension. Which of the following is the most appropriate first step in evaluation?

a. Serum testosterone
b. Serum gonadotropin
c. Information about libido and morning erections
d. Papaverine injection

202. A 90-year-old male complains of hip and back pain. He has also developed headaches, hearing loss, and tinnitus. On physical exam the skull appears enlarged, with prominent superficial veins. There is marked kyphosis, and the bones of the leg appear deformed. Plasma alkaline phosphatase is elevated. A skull x-ray shows sharply demarcated lucencies in the frontal, parietal, and occipital bones. X-rays of the hip show thickening of the pelvic brim. Which of the following is the most likely diagnosis?

a. Multiple myeloma
b. Paget's disease
c. Hypercalcemia
d. Metastatic bone disease

203. A 48-year-old female presents to your office on suggestion from a urologist. She has had three episodes of kidney stones. She is taking no medications. She tells you that at a recent health fair a screening heel densitometry indicated that she might have osteoporosis. She is very concerned that something else is going on and wants you to run some more tests. Within the past month, she has had basic lab work consisting of the following:

Na: 139
K: 4.2
HCO_3: 25
Cl: 101
BUN: 19
Creatinine: 1.1
Ca: 10.4

Which of the following tests will confirm the most likely diagnosis?

a. Thyroid function profile
b. The iPTH test
c. Liver function tests
d. 24-h urine calcium

204. A patient comes to your office for a new-patient visit. He has recently moved from Kansas City to Oklahoma City due to a job promotion. His last annual exam was 1 month prior to his move. He received a letter from his primary physician stating that laboratory workup had revealed an elevated alkaline phosphatase and that he needed to have this evaluated by a physician in his new location. On questioning, his only complaint is pain below the knee that has not gotten better with over-the-counter medications. The pain increases with standing. He denies trauma to the area. On exam you note slight warmth just below the knee, no deformity or effusion of the knee joint, and the patient has full ROM of the knee without pain. You order an x-ray, which shows cortical thickening of the superior fibula and sclerotic changes. Laboratory evaluation shows an elevated alkaline phosphatase of 297 with an otherwise normal metabolic panel. Which of the following is the treatment of choice for this patient?

a. Observation
b. Nonsteroidal anti-inflammatory
c. Calcitonin or bisphosphonates
d. Interferon α

205. A 30-year-old female complains of fatigue, constipation, and weight gain. There is no prior history of neck surgery or radiation. Her voice is hoarse and her skin is dry. Serum TSH is elevated and T_4 is low. Which of the following is the most likely cause of these findings?

a. Autoimmune disease
b. Postablative hypothyroidism
c. Pituitary hypofunction
d. Thyroid carcinoma

206. A 40-year-old alcoholic male is being treated for tuberculosis, but he has not been compliant with his medications. He complains of increasing weakness and fatigue. He appears to have lost weight, and his blood pressure is 80/50 mmHg. There is increased pigmentation over the elbows. Cardiac exam is normal. Which of the following is the best next step in evaluation?

a. CBC with iron and iron-binding capacity
b. Erythrocyte sedimentation rate
c. Early morning serum cortisol and cosyntropin stimulation
d. Blood cultures

207. A family brings their 82-year-old grandmother to the emergency room stating that they cannot care for her anymore. They tell you, "She has just been getting sicker and sicker." Now she stays in bed and won't eat due to stomach pain. She has diarrhea most of the time and can barely make it to the bathroom because of her weakness. Her symptoms have been worsening over the past year, but she refused to see a doctor. On exam the patient is talkative and denies symptoms of depression. There are orthostatic changes on exam. Heart and lung exam is normal. Skin exam reveals a bronze coloring to the elbows and palmar creases. What laboratory abnormality would you expect to find in this patient?

a. Low serum Na^+
b. Low serum K^+
c. Low serum Na^+ and high serum K^+
d. Low serum K^+

208. A 47-year-old male homeless man presents to the indigent clinic. He was recently discharged from the hospital with a diagnosis of Addison's disease (primary adrenal insufficiency). The patient states that the doctor at the hospital told him if he did not take medication he might die. He reports that he left his prescriptions and discharge instructions on the bus that took him to a shelter near the hospital. He asks you to give him new prescriptions. You get his medical records faxed over from the hospital and, after reviewing them, agree with his diagnosis of Addison's disease. Which of the following is the treatment of choice for this patient?

a. Hydrocortisone once per day
b. Hydrocortisone twice per day plus fludrocortisone
c. Hydrocortisone only during periods of stress
d. Daily ACTH

209. A 60-year-old woman comes to the emergency room in a coma. The patient's temperature is 90°F. She is bradycardic. Her thyroid gland is enlarged. There is bilateral hyporeflexia. Which of the following is the best next step in management?

a. Await results of T_4, TSH
b. Obtain T_4, TSH; begin thyroid hormone and glucocorticoid
c. Begin rapid rewarming
d. Obtain CT scan of the head

210. A 19-year-old with insulin-dependent diabetes mellitus is taking 30 units of NPH insulin each morning and 15 units at night. Because of persistent morning glycosuria with some ketonuria, the evening dose is increased to 20 units. This worsens the morning glycosuria, and now moderate ketones are noted in urine. The patient complains of sweats and headaches at night. Which of the following is the most appropriate next step in management?

a. Increase the evening dose of insulin
b. Increase the morning dose of insulin
c. Switch from human NPH to pork insulin
d. Obtain blood sugar levels between 2:00 and 5:00 A.M.

211. A 30-year-old woman is found to have a low serum thyroxine level after being evaluated for fatigue. Five years ago she was treated for Graves' disease with radioactive iodine. Which of the following is the diagnostic test of choice?

a. Serum TSH
b. Serum T_3
c. TRH stimulation test
d. Radioactive iodine uptake

212. A 25-year-old woman is admitted for hypertensive crisis. In the hospital, blood pressure is labile and responds poorly to antihypertensive therapy. The patient complains of palpitations and apprehension. Her past medical history shows that she developed hypotension during an operation for appendicitis.

Hct: 49% (37–48)
WBC: 11×10^3 mm (4.3–10.8)
Plasma glucose: 160 mg/dL (75–115)
Plasma calcium: 11 mg/dL (9–10.5)

Which of the following is the most likely diagnosis?

a. Pheochromocytoma
b. Renal artery stenosis
c. Essential hypertension
d. Insulin-dependent diabetes mellitus

213. The patient pictured below complains of persistent headache. Which of the following is her most likely visual field defect?

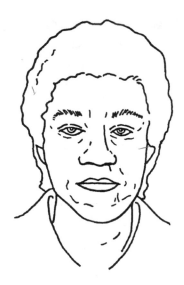

a. Bitemporal hemianopsia
b. Unilateral blindness
c. Left homonymous hemianopsia
d. Right homonymous hemianopsia

214. A patient with small cell carcinoma of the lung develops lethargy. Serum electrolytes are drawn and show a serum sodium of 118 mg/L. There is no evidence of edema, orthostatic hypotension, or dehydration. Urine is concentrated with an osmolality of 320 mmol/kg. Serum BUN, creatinine, and glucose are within normal range. Which of the following is the next appropriate step?

a. Normal saline infusion
b. Diuresis
c. Fluid restriction
d. Tetracycline

215. The 40-year-old woman shown below complains of weakness and amenorrhea. She has hypertension and diabetes mellitus. The clinical findings may be explained by which of the following?

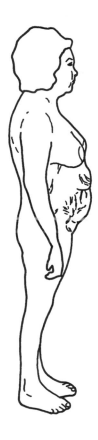

a. Pituitary tumor
b. Adrenal tumor
c. Ectopic ACTH production
d. Any of the above

216. The patient pictured below presents with gynecomastia and infertility. On exam, he has small, firm testes. Which of the following is correct?

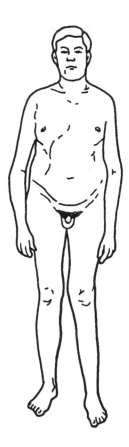

a. The patient is likely to have low levels of gonadotropins
b. The patient has Turner syndrome
c. His most likely karyotype is 47 XXY
d. The patient will have normal sperm count and testosterone level

217. A 52-year-old man complains of impotence. On physical examination, he has an elevated jugular venous pressure, S_3 gallop, and hepatomegaly. He also appears tanned, with pigmentation along joint folds. His left knee is swollen and tender. The plasma glucose is 250 mg/dL, and liver enzymes are elevated. Which of the following studies will help establish the diagnosis?

a. Detection of nocturnal penile tumescence
b. Determination of iron saturation
c. Determination of serum copper
d. Detection of hepatitis B surface antigen
e. Echocardiography

218. A 30-year-old man is evaluated for a thyroid nodule. The patient reports that his father died from thyroid cancer and that a brother had a history of recurrent renal stones. Blood calcitonin concentration is 2000 pg/mL (normal is less than 100); serum calcium and phosphate levels are normal. Before referring the patient to a surgeon, the physician should do which of the following?

a. Obtain a liver scan
b. Perform a calcium infusion test
c. Measure urinary catecholamines
d. Administer suppressive doses of thyroxine and measure levels of thyroid-stimulating hormone
e. Treat the patient with radioactive iodine

219. A 32-year-old woman has a 3-year history of oligomenorrhea that has progressed to amenorrhea during the past year. She has observed loss of breast fullness, reduced hip measurements, acne, increased body hair, and deepening of her voice. Physical examination reveals frontal balding, clitoral hypertrophy, and a male escutcheon. Urinary free cortisol and dehydroepiandrosterone sulfate (DHEAS) are normal. Her plasma testosterone level is 6 ng/mL (normal is 0.2 to 0.8). Which of the following is the most likely diagnosis?

a. Cushing syndrome
b. Arrhenoblastoma
c. Polycystic ovary syndrome
d. Granulosa-theca cell tumor

220. A 54-year-old man who has had a Billroth II procedure for peptic ulcer disease now presents with abdominal pain and is found to have recurrent ulcer disease. The physician is considering this patient's illness to be secondary either to a retained antrum or to a gastrinoma. Which of the following tests would best differentiate the two conditions?

a. Random gastrin level
b. Determination of 24-h acid production
c. Serum calcium level
d. Secretin infusion
e. Insulin-induced hypoglycemia

221. A 55-year-old woman who has a history of severe depression and who had radical mastectomy for carcinoma of the breast 1 year previously develops polyuria, nocturia, and excessive thirst. Laboratory values are as follows:

Serum electrolytes: Na⁻ 149 meq/L; K⁻ 3.6 meq/L
Serum calcium: 9.5 mg/dL
Blood glucose: 110 mg/dL
Blood urea nitrogen: 30 mg/dL
Urine osmolality: 150 mOsm/kg

Which of the following is the most likely diagnosis?

a. Psychogenic polydipsia
b. Renal glycosuria
c. Hypercalciuria
d. Diabetes insipidus
e. Inappropriate antidiuretic hormone syndrome

222. A 30-year-old nursing student presents with confusion, sweating, hunger, and fatigue. Blood sugar is noted to be 40 mg/dL. The patient has no history of diabetes mellitus, although her sister is an insulin-dependent diabetic. The patient has had several similar episodes over the past year, all occurring just prior to reporting for work in the early morning. On this evaluation, the patient is found to have high insulin levels and a low C peptide level. Which of the following is the most likely diagnosis?

a. Reactive hypoglycemia
b. Early diabetes mellitus
c. Factitious hypoglycemia
d. Insulinoma

223. A 60-year-old male presents for follow-up of hyperlipidemia and hypertension. Laboratory evaluation reveals well-controlled hyperlipidemia with a total cholesterol of 176 and LDL 104. However, liver function testing reveals an elevated alkaline phosphatase at 250. You fractionate the alkaline phosphatase and the skeletal component is elevated. You tell the patient he may have Paget's disease. The cause of this disease is which of the following?

a. Endocrinopathy
b. Viral infection
c. Malignancy
d. Unknown

DIRECTIONS: Each group of questions below consists of lettered options followed by a set of numbered items. For each numbered item, select the **one** lettered option with which it is **most** closely associated. Each lettered option may be used once, more than once, or not at all.

Questions 224–226

Select the most likely disease process for the clinical syndromes described.

a. Acromegaly
b. Prolactin-secreting adenoma
c. Cushing's disease
d. Empty sella syndrome
e. TSH-secreting adenoma
f. Diabetes insipidus

224. A 30-year-old woman has cervical fat pad, purple striae, and hirsutism.

225. A nonpregnant woman has bitemporal hemianopsia, irregular menses, and galactorrhea.

226. An obese hypertensive woman has chronic headaches and normal pituitary function.

Questions 227–229

Match each symptom or sign with the appropriate disease.

a. Subacute thyroiditis
b. Graves' disease
c. Surreptitious hyperthyroidism
d. Multinodular goiter
e. Thyroid nodule

227. Patient presents with weakness, tremor, heat intolerance; skin is raised and thickened with peau d'orange appearance.

228. Male nursing assistant presents with weakness and tremor; there are no ophthalmopathy or skin lesions; RAIU shows subnormal values; T_4 is elevated.

229. A 20-year-old presents after recent upper respiratory infection. She complains of neck pain. The thyroid is tender; erythrocyte sedimentation rate is elevated; patient exhibits heat intolerance.

Endocrinology and Metabolic Disease

Answers

190. The answer is b. (*Stobo, pp 328–329.*) This obese patient on oral hypoglycemics has developed hyperglycemia and lethargy during an upper respiratory infection. Hyperosmolar nonketotic states that occur in type 2 diabetes can be fatal. When severe hyperglycemia and dehydration increase serum osmolarity above 380 mOsm/L, lethargy or coma occurs. Serum osmolarity is measured by the formula:

$$\frac{\text{Plasma glucose}}{18} + 2 \, (\text{serum Na}^+ + \text{K}^+) + \frac{\text{blood urea nitrogen}}{2.8}$$

This patient's serum osmolality is as follows:

$$\frac{900}{18} + 2 \, (138) + \frac{84}{2.8} = 50 + 276 + 30 = 356$$

Thus the serum osmolality is greater than 350 mOsm/kg. As can be seen from the equation, osmolarity depends mostly on the concentration of sodium. Serum osmolarity will rise significantly when dehydration prevents the dilution of serum sodium that might otherwise occur with hyperglycemia. Hyperosmolarity reflects both hyperglycemia and severe dehydration with hypernatremia. The serum bicarbonate is too high to be consistent with diabetic ketoacidosis. The hyponatremia is related to hyperglycemia. SIADH could not be diagnosed in this clinical setting. Patients with SIADH are not dehydrated but have an inappropriate excretion of ADH that leads to hyponatremia and water retention. The patient's diabetes likely went out of control due to infection. There is no clinical evidence for meningitis.

191. The answer is a. (*Kasper, p 2161.*) The primary treatment for hyperosmolar nonketotic states is fluid replacement, usually normal saline over the first 2 to 3 h. Hypotonic saline may be given for severe hypernatremia or congestive heart failure. Hyperglycemia can be corrected slowly. The patient is not acidotic and would not require bicarbonate treatment (used in severe DKA when pH is less than 7.0). The patient's serum potassium is in the normal range and would not be expected to fall rapidly, but should be monitored.

192. The answer is b. *(Kasper, p 2171.)* The classification of diabetes mellitus has changed to emphasize the process that leads to hyperglycemia. Type 2 DM is a group of heterogeneous disorders characterized by insulin resistance, impaired secretion of insulin, and increased glucose production. *Medical nutrition therapy* (MNT) is a term now used to describe the best possible coordination of calorie intake, weight loss, and exercise. It emphasizes modification of risk factors for hypertension and hyperlipidemia, not just weight loss and calorie restriction. In this type 2 patient, medical nutrition therapy that includes dietary modification, weight loss, and exercise is the first intervention. Blood glucose control should be reevaluated after 3 to 4 weeks. If target blood sugar is not met, pharmacotherapy should be initiated.

193. The answer is b. *(Kasper, pp 2113–2117.)* This patient has clinical symptoms of thyrotoxicosis. Most patients with thyrotoxicosis have increases in total and free concentrations of T_3 and T_4. (Some may have isolated T_3 or T_4 increases.) Most thyrotoxicosis results in suppression of pituitary TSH secretion, so low TSH levels can also confirm the diagnosis.

194. The answer is a. *(Kasper, pp 2113–2117.)* This patient has Graves' disease, which accounts for 60 to 80% of all thyrotoxicosis. In addition to thyrotoxicosis, this patient has orbitopathy as well as the characteristic dermopathy of Graves' disease, called *pretibial myxedema*. Graves' disease is an autoimmune phenomenon. The extrathyroidal manifestations of the diseases are due to immunologically activated fibroblasts in extraocular muscles and skin. Toxic multinodular goiter produces thyrotoxicosis caused by benign, functionally autonomous tumors. The thyroid gland is usually appreciated as a palpably nodular goiter. Toxic multinodular goiter would not produce the proptosis or dermopathy of Graves' disease. Subacute thyroiditis (de Quervain's) is probably caused by a viral infection. It produces a transient hyperthyroidism followed by hypothyroidism. The thyroid gland is tender.

195. The answer is a. *(Kasper, pp 2116–2117.)* Antithyroid drugs are considered by most to be the treatment of choice in a patient with Graves' disease when the underlying illness may remit. Surgical thyroidectomy is usually reserved for those with thyroid malignancy or thyrotoxic pregnant women who have had severe side effects to medication. Surgery complications include hypoparathyroidism and recurrent laryngeal nerve injury. Iodine 131 has been used successfully in Graves' disease and is a reasonable option if the patient is not pregnant or breastfeeding. However, it often causes permanent hypothyroidism. It has also been reported to worsen ophthalmopathy in some patients. The treatment of choice is an oral agent, propylthiouracil. Propylthiouracil is chosen in cases such as this due to low transplacental transfer. Radioactive iodine would not be used in a pregnant female but may be used in women desiring pregnancy if given prior to 6 months of conception. As this patient is currently attempting conception, the benefit of radioactive iodine treatment would not outweigh the risk. Thyroid surgery is reserved for patients who do not respond to oral agents or radioactive iodine. Oral corticosteroids are not used in Graves' disease.

196. The answer is c. (*Kasper, pp 2138–2140.*) The patient has diastolic hypertension with associated hypokalemia. She is not taking diuretics. There is no edema on physical exam. Excessive inappropriate aldosterone production will produce a hypertension with hypokalemia syndrome. Hypersecretion of aldosterone increases distal tubular exchange of sodium for potassium with progressive depletion of body potassium. The hypertension is due to increased sodium absorption. Very low plasma renin that fails to increase with appropriate stimulus (such as volume depletion) and hypersecretion of aldosterone suggest the diagnosis of primary hyperaldosteronism. Suppressed renin activity occurs in about 25% of hypertensive patients with essential hypertension. Lack of suppression of aldosterone is also necessary to diagnose primary aldosteronism. High aldosterone levels that are not suppressed by saline loading prove that there is a primary inappropriate secretion of aldosterone. A 24-h urine for free cortisol would be used in the workup of a patient with Cushing syndrome. Urinary metanephrine is a screening test for pheochromocytoma.

197. The answer is a. (*Kasper, pp 2110–2113.*) Once hypothyroidism is diagnosed by clinical features and TSH and free T_4 measurements, etiology can be confirmed by measuring the presence of autoantibody—particularly thyroid peroxidase (TPO), which is present in 90 to 95% of patients with autoimmune hypothyroidism. Biopsy by fine needle aspirate can confirm the diagnosis but is not necessary in most cases.

198. The answer is d. *(Kasper, p 2126.)* Palpable thyroid nodules are common, occurring in about 5% of all adults. Thyroid fine needle biopsy now plays a central role in the differential diagnosis of thyroid nodules. If the TSH is normal, as it is in this patient, then fine needle aspirate biopsy is indicated and will distinguish cysts from benign lesions or neoplasms. In about 14% of such cases, biopsy will be suspicious or diagnostic for malignancy and surgery will be necessary. Thyroid scan can show a hot nodule, which would be reassuring that the nodule is benign; however, a biopsy would be necessary for cold nodules. Thyroid sonography seldom can rule out malignancy in palpable nodules.

199. The answer is d. *(Kasper, p 2171.)* An active lifestyle and a good exercise program can prevent the complications of diabetes. Benefits include blood pressure control, reduction in body fat, weight loss, and increased insulin sensitivity. However, there are pitfalls to such a program. Some forms of exercise might jeopardize adequate foot care, and foot exam becomes particularly important in the patient who is doing weight-bearing exercise. Exercise can induce hypoglycemia by potentiating insulin action; this is particularly true in the type 1 diabetic. Diabetics who have risk factors for cardiovascular disease, such as hypertension and hyperlipidemia, should undergo an exercise stress test prior to engaging in a rigorous exercise program. This is important because asymptomatic cardiovascular disease is more common in diabetics.

200. The answer is c. *(Kasper, p 2171.)* In order to reduce plasma cholesterol and decrease the risk of vascular disease, fat intake should be moderated, with less than 10% of total caloric intake being saturated fat. Caloric distribution does not restrict or decrease carbohydrates. Use of caloric sweeteners, including sucrose, is acceptable as long as it is matched to insulin demand. Dietary protein should provide 10 to 20% of total calories. In patients with diabetic nephropathy, reducing dietary protein to 10% is often recommended. Caloric intake is not consistent from day to day but is matched with level of activity.

201. The answer is c. *(Kasper, pp 272–273.)* The first step in the evaluation of impotence is a complete and detailed history, including libido and ability to attain erection unrelated to sexual intercourse. Loss of all erectile function suggests an organic cause for the disease. In this patient, impotence may be the result of depression from the antihypertensive agent or a direct effect of the beta blocker on sexual performance. Diabetes may cause impotence as an effect on penile blood supply or parasympathetic nervous system function. A decrease in libido would suggest testosterone deficiency. Serum testosterone should then be measured, and, if low, serum gonadotropins should be measured. In a diabetic with claudication or abnormal femoral pulses, injection of papaverine into the corpora cavernosa can test vascular insufficiency as the cause of impotence. A normal response is an erection within 10 min.

202. The answer is b. (*Kasper, pp 2279–2281.*) This patient has widespread Paget's disease of bone. Excessive resorption of bone is followed by replacement of normal marrow with dense, trabecular, disorganized bone. Hearing loss and tinnitus are due to direct involvement of the ossicles of the inner ear. Plasma alkaline phosphatase levels represent increased bone turnover. Neither myeloma or metastatic bone disease would result in bony deformity such as skull enlargement. Alkaline phosphatase is a marker of bone formation and does not rise in pure lytic lesions such as multiple myeloma.

203. The answer is b. (*Kasper, pp 2254, 2268–2278.*) Sequelae of hyperparathyroidism include renal stones. Secondary causes such as osteoporosis should definitely be considered in this premenopausal female. Hyperparathyroidism, hyperthyroidism, chronic oral steroid use, vitamin D deficiency, Cushing's syndrome, and celiac sprue are some of the causes of secondary osteoporosis.

204. The answer is c. (*Kasper, pp 2281–2282.*) Most patients with Paget's disease do not require treatment, as they are asymptomatic. Bone pain, hearing loss, bony deformity, congestive heart failure, hypercalcemia, and repeated fractures are all indications for specific therapy beyond just the symptomatic relief of nonsteroidal anti-inflammatory agents. Calcitonin restores normal bone modeling. Bisphosphonates bind to hydroxyapatite crystals to decrease bone turnover. Bisphosphonates are now generally recommended as the treatment of choice. Newer bisphosphonates such as alendronate and risedronate have replaced editronate because they are more potent and do not produce mineralization defects. Subcutaneous injectable calcitonin is still used in patients who cannot tolerate the GI side effects of bisphosphonates.

205. The answer is a. (*Kasper, pp 2110–2113.*) This patient presents with classic features of hypothyroidism. Autoimmune thyroiditis usually occurs in women, has a genetic component, and is associated with other autoimmune conditions. Autoimmune thyroiditis may be present with a goiter (Hashimoto's thyroiditis) or with minimal residual thyroid tissue (atrophic thyroiditis). Once hypothyroidism is diagnosed by clinical features and TSH and free T_4 measurements, etiology can be confirmed by measuring the presence of autoantibody—particularly thyroid peroxidase (TPO), which is present in 90 to 95% of patients with autoimmune hypothyroidism. Biopsy by fine needle aspirate can confirm the diagnosis but is not necessary in most cases.

206. The answer is c. (*Kasper, pp 2141–2143.*) This patient's symptoms of weakness, fatigue, and weight loss in combination with signs of hypotension and extensor hyperpigmentation are all consistent with Addison's disease (adrenal insufficiency). Tuberculosis can involve the adrenal glands and result in adrenal insufficiency. Measurement of serum cortisol baseline and then stimulation with ACTH will confirm the clinical suspicion. The ACTH stimulation test is used to determine the adrenal reserve capacity for steroid production. Cortisol response is measured 60 min after cosyntropin is given intramuscularly or intravenously.

207. The answer is c. (*Kasper, pp 2141–2143.*) This patient's presentation is consistent with a diagnosis of adrenal insufficiency (Addison's disease). Hyponatremia is due to loss of sodium in the urine (aldosterone deficiency) and movement of sodium intracellularly. Extravascular sodium loss causes hypotension. Hyperkalemia is due to aldosterone deficiency, impaired glomerular filtration, and acidosis.

208. The answer is b. (*Kasper, pp 2141–2143.*) Hydrocortisone is the mainstay of treatment. Two-thirds of the dose is taken in the morning and one-third at night in order to approach normal diurnal variation. The recommended dose is 20 to 30 mg/d. The mineralocorticoid component of adrenal hormones also needs to be replaced. Fludrocortisone is given at a dosage of 0.05 to 0.1 mg/d. During periods of intercurrent stress or illness, higher doses of both glucocorticoid and mineralocorticoid are required.

209. The answer is b. *(Kasper, pp 2112–2113.)* The clinical concern in this patient is myxedema coma. Once this diagnosis is considered, treatment must be started, as it is a medical emergency. Treatment is initiated; should lab results not support the diagnosis, then treatment would be stopped. An intravenous bolus of thyroxine is given (300 to 500 mcg), followed by daily intravenous doses. Glucocorticoids are given concomitantly. Intravenous fluids are also needed; rewarming should be accompanied slowly, so as not to precipitate cardiac arrhythmias. If alveolar ventilation is compromised, then intubation may also be necessary.

210. The answer is d. *(Stein, p 1861.)* Episodic hypoglycemia at night is followed by rebound hyperglycemia. This condition, called the Somogyi phenomenon, develops in response to excessive insulin administration. An adrenergic response to hypoglycemia results in increased glycogenolysis, gluconeogenesis, and diminished glucose uptake by peripheral tissues. After hypoglycemia is documented, the insulin dosages are slowly reduced.

211. The answer is a. *(Stein, pp 1808–1811.)* TSH levels are always increased in patients with untreated hypothyroidism (from primary thyroid disease) and would be the test of choice in this patient. Serum T_3 is not sensitive for hypothyroidism. The TRH stimulation test is used to assess pituitary reserve of thyroid-stimulating hormone. A decreased RAIU is of limited value because of the low value for the lower limit of normal. In goitrous hypothyroidism, the RAIU may even be increased.

212. The answer is a. *(Kasper, pp 2149–2150.)* A hypertensive crisis in this young woman suggests a secondary cause of hypertension. In the setting of palpitations, apprehension, and hyperglycemia, pheochromocytoma should be considered. Pheochromocytomas are derived from the adrenal medulla. They are capable of producing and secreting catecholamines. Unexplained hypertension associated with surgery or trauma may also suggest the disease. Clinical symptoms are the result of catecholamine secretion. For example, the patient's hyperglycemia is a result of a catecholamine effect of insulin suppression and stimulation of hepatic glucose output. Hypercalcemia has been attributed to ectopic secretion of parathormone-related protein. Renal artery stenosis can cause severe hypertension but would not explain the systemic symptoms or laboratory abnormalities in this case.

213. The answer is a. (*Kasper, pp 2090–2091.*) The patient shows excessive growth of soft tissue that has resulted in coarsening of facial features, prognathism, and frontal bossing—all characteristic of acromegaly. This growth hormone–secreting pituitary tumor will result in bitemporal hemianopsia when the tumor impinges on the optic chiasm, which lies just above the sella turcica.

214. The answer is c. (*Kasper, pp 2102–2103.*) The patient described has hyponatremia, normovolemia, and concentrated urine. These features are sufficient to make a diagnosis of inappropriate antidiuretic hormone secretion. Inappropriate ADH secretion occurs, in some cases, due to ectopic production by neoplastic tissue. Treatment necessitates restriction of fluid intake. A negative water balance results in a rise in serum Na^+ and serum osmolality and symptom improvement. This syndrome can occur as a side effect of many drugs or from carcinoma, head trauma, infections, neurologic diseases, or stroke.

215. The answer is d. (*Kasper, pp 2092–2093.*) The clinical findings all suggest an excess production of cortisol by the adrenal gland. Hypertension, truncal obesity, and abdominal striae are common physical findings. The process responsible for continued excess could be any of those listed—an ACTH-secreting pituitary tumor, an ectopic ACTH-producing neoplasm, or a primary adrenal tumor.

216. The answer is c. (*Kasper, pp 2214–2216.*) The picture of infertility, gynecomastia, and tall stature is consistent with Klinefelter syndrome and an XXY karyotype. The patient has abnormal gonadal development with hyalinized testes that result in low testosterone levels and elevated levels of gonadotropin. Turner syndrome refers to the 45 XO karyotype that results in abnormal sexual development in a female.

217. The answer is b. (*Kasper, pp 2298–2302.*) Iron overload should be considered among patients who present with any one or a combination of the following: hepatomegaly, weakness, pigmentation, atypical arthritis, diabetes, impotence, unexplained chronic abdominal pain, or cardiomyopathy. Excessive alcohol intake increases the diagnostic probability. Diagnostic suspicions should be particularly high when the family history is positive for similar clinical findings. The most frequent cause of iron overload is a common genetic disorder known as (idiopathic) hemochromatosis. Secondary iron storage problems can occur in a variety of anemias. The most practical screening test is the determination of serum iron, transferrin saturation, and plasma ferritin. Plasma ferritin values above 300 ng/mL in males and 200 ng/mL in females suggest increased iron stores. Genetic screening is now used to assess which patients are at risk for severe fibrosis of the liver. Definitive diagnosis can be established by liver biopsy. Determination of serum copper is needed when Wilson's disease is the probable cause of hepatic abnormalities. The clinical picture here is inconsistent with that diagnosis. Nocturnal penile tumescence and echocardiogram can confirm clinical findings but will not help to establish the diagnosis.

218. The answer is c. (*Kasper, pp 2234–2236.*) For the patient described, the markedly increased calcitonin levels indicate the diagnosis of medullary carcinoma of the thyroid. In view of the family history, the patient most likely has multiple endocrine neoplasia (MEN) type II, which includes medullary carcinoma of the thyroid gland, pheochromocytoma, and parathyroid hyperplasia. Pheochromocytoma may exist without sustained hypertension, as indicated by excessive urinary catecholamines. Before thyroid surgery is performed on this patient, a pheochromocytoma must be ruled out through urinary catecholamine determinations; the presence of such a tumor might expose him to a hypertensive crisis during surgery. The entire thyroid gland must be removed because foci of parafollicular cell hyperplasia, a premalignant lesion, may be scattered throughout the gland. Successful removal of the medullary carcinoma can be monitored with serum calcitonin levels. Hyperparathyroidism, while unlikely in this patient, is probably present in his brother. Hypoparathyroidism is unlikely with a normal serum calcium level.

219. The answer is b. (*Kasper, pp 555–556.*) The symptoms of masculinization (e.g., alopecia, deepening of voice, clitoral hypertrophy) in the patient presented in the question are characteristic of active androgen-producing tumors. Such extreme virilization is very rarely observed in polycystic ovary syndrome or in Cushing syndrome; moreover, the presence of normal cortisol and markedly elevated plasma testosterone levels indicates an ovarian rather than adrenal cause of the findings. Arrhenoblastomas are the most common androgen-producing ovarian tumors. Their incidence is highest during the reproductive years. Composed of varying proportions of Leydig's and Sertoli cells, they are generally benign. In contrast to arrhenoblastomas, granulosa-theca cell tumors produce feminization, not virilization.

220. The answer is d. *(Kasper, pp 1758–1759, 2227.)* The diagnosis of gastrinoma should be considered in all patients with recurrent ulcers after surgical correction for peptic ulcer disease, ulcers in the distal duodenum or jejunum, ulcer disease associated with diarrhea, or evidence suggestive of the multiple endocrine neoplasia (MEN) type I (familial association of pituitary, parathyroid, and pancreatic tumors) in ulcer patients. Because basal serum gastrin and basal acid production may both be normal or only slightly elevated in patients with gastrinomas, provocative tests may be needed for diagnosis. Both the secretin and calcium infusion tests are used; a paradoxical increase in serum gastrin concentration is seen in response to both infusions in patients with gastrinomas. In contrast, other conditions associated with hypergastrinemia, such as duodenal ulcers, retained antrum, gastric outlet obstruction, antral G cell hyperplasia, and pernicious anemia, will respond with either no change or a decrease in serum gastrin.

221. The answer is d. *(Kasper, pp 2098–2100.)* Metastatic tumors rarely cause diabetes insipidus, but of the tumors that may cause it, carcinoma of the breast is by far the most common. In this patient, the diagnosis of diabetes insipidus is suggested by hypernatremia and low urine osmolality. Psychogenic polydipsia is an unlikely diagnosis since serum sodium is usually mildly reduced in this condition. Renal glycosuria would be expected to induce a higher urine osmolality than this patient has because of the osmotic effect of glucose. While nephrocalcinosis secondary to hypercalcemia may produce polyuria, hypercalciuria does not. Finally, the findings of inappropriate antidiuretic hormone syndrome are the opposite of those observed in diabetes insipidus and thus are incompatible with the clinical picture in this patient.

222. The answer is c. *(Kasper, pp 2182–2184.)* This clinical picture and laboratory results suggest factitious hypoglycemia caused by self-administration of insulin. The diagnosis should be suspected in health care workers, patients or family members with diabetes, and others who have a history of malingering. Patients present with symptoms of hypoglycemia and low plasma glucose levels. Insulin levels will be high, but without a concomitant rise in C peptide. Endogenous hyperinsulinism, such as would be seen with an insulinoma, would result in elevated plasma insulin concentrations (>36 pmol/L) and elevated C peptide levels (>0.2 mmol/L). C peptide is derived from the breakdown of proinsulin, which is produced endogenously; thus C peptide will not rise in the patient who develops hypoglycemia from exogenous insulin. Reactive hypoglycemia occurs after meals and is self-limited. A rapid postprandial rise in glucose may induce a brisk insulin response that causes transient hypoglycemia hours later. It may be associated with gastric or intestinal surgery.

223. The answer is d. *(Kasper, pp 2279–2281.)* The cause of Paget's disease remains unknown. Some intranuclear inclusions resemble the nucleocapsids of viruses. Measles and respiratory syncytial virus mRNA appears similar to mRNA found in nucleocapsids. No known endocrinopathy has been suggested, and Paget's disease does not involve malignant cells. There is increasing interest in a genetic predisposition for the disease, and some kindreds have an autosomal dominant inheritance pattern.

224–226. The answers are 224-c, 225-b, 226-d. *(Kasper, pp 2079, 2085–2086, 2093.)* Cushing's disease produces hypercortisolism secondary to excessive excretion of pituitary ACTH. It often affects women in their childbearing years. Cervical fat pad, purple striae, and hirsutism are characteristic features, as well as muscle wasting, easy bruising, amenorrhea, and psychiatric disturbances. Prolactinoma, or prolactin-secreting adenoma, may cause bitemporal hemianopsia—as all pituitary tumors can. Galactorrhea (lactation not associated with pregnancy) and irregular menses or amenorrhea are the clinical clues. Serum prolactin levels are usually over 250 ng/mL, often distinguishing them from other causes of hyperprolactinemia such as renal failure. Empty sella syndrome is enlargement of the sella turcica from CSF pressure compressing the pituitary gland. It is likely to occur in obese, hypertensive women. There are no focal findings. Some patients have chronic headaches; others are asymptomatic.

MRI will distinguish this syndrome from a pituitary tumor. These patients have normal pituitary function, the rim of pituitary tissue being fully functional.

227–229. The answers are 227-b, 228-c, 229-a. *(Kasper, pp 2213–2118.)* Symptoms of hyperthyroidism with skin involvement characteristic of pretibial myxedema suggest Graves' disease. Skin and eye involvement in association with hyperthyroid symptoms do not occur in hyperthyroidism other than Graves' disease. Surreptitious hyperthyroidism can occur in health care workers who have access to thyroid hormone. Classic symptoms of hyperthyroidism occur and the serum T_4 is elevated. Radioactive iodine uptake would show subnormal values, as there is no increased thyroid uptake in the gland itself. The thyroid gland is not palpable. A tender thyroid gland and elevated ESR make subacute thyroiditis a likely diagnosis. Hyperthyroid symptoms are common early in the illness.

Gastroenterology

Questions

DIRECTIONS: Each item below contains a question followed by suggested responses. Select the **one best** response to each question.

230. A 35-year-old alcoholic male is admitted for nausea, vomiting, and abdominal pain that radiates to the back. Which of the following laboratory values suggests a poor prognosis in this patient?

a. Elevated serum lipase
b. Elevated serum amylase
c. Leukocytosis of 20,000/μm ·
d. Diastolic blood pressure greater than 90 mmHg

231. A 40-year-old cigarette smoker complains of epigastric pain, well localized, nonradiating, and described as burning. The pain is partially relieved by eating. There is no weight loss. He has not used nonsteroidal anti-inflammatory agents. The pain has gradually worsened over several months. Which of the following is the most sensitive way to make a specific diagnosis?

a. Barium x-ray
b. Endoscopy ·
c. Serologic test for *Helicobacter pylori*
d. Serum gastrin

232. A 56-year-old woman becomes the chief financial officer of a large company and, several months thereafter, develops upper abdominal pain that she ascribes to stress. She takes an over-the-counter antacid with temporary benefit. She uses no other medications. One night she awakens with nausea and vomits a large volume of coffee grounds–like material; she becomes weak and diaphoretic. Upon hospitalization, she is found to have an actively bleeding duodenal ulcer. What is the likelihood that *Helicobacter pylori* will be found on biopsy specimens?

a. 5%
b. 10%
c. 70%
d. 100%

233. A 36-year-old man presents for a well-patient exam. He gives a history that, over the past 20 years, he has had three episodes of abdominal pain and hematemesis, the most recent of which occurred several years ago. He was told that an ulcer was seen on a barium upper GI radiograph. You obtain a serum assay for *Helicobacter pylori* IgG, which is positive. What is the most effective regimen to eradicate this organism?

a. Omeprazole 20 mg PO daily for 6 weeks
b. Ranitidine 300 mg PO qhs for 6 weeks
c. Omeprazole 20 mg bid, amoxicillin 1000 mg bid, clarithromycin 500 mg bid for 14 days
d. Pepto-Bismol and metronidazole bid for 7 days

234. A 70-year-old male presents with a complaint of fatigue. There is no history of alcohol abuse or liver disease; the patient is taking no medications. Scleral icterus is noted on physical exam. There is no evidence for chronic liver disease on physical exam, and the liver and spleen are non-palpable. The patient has a normocytic, normochromic anemia. Urinalysis shows bilirubinuria with absent urine urobilinogen. Serum bilirubin is 12 mg/dL, AST and ALT are in normal range, and alkaline phosphatase is 300 U/L (3 times normal). Which of the following is the best next step in evaluation?

a. Ultrasound or CT scan
b. Hepatitis profile
c. Reticulocyte count
d. Family history for hemochromatosis

235. A 58-year-old white man complains of intermittent rectal bleeding and, at the time of colonoscopy, is found to have internal hemorrhoids and the lesion shown at the splenic flexure. Pathology shows tubulovillous changes. Repeat colonoscopy should be recommended at what interval?

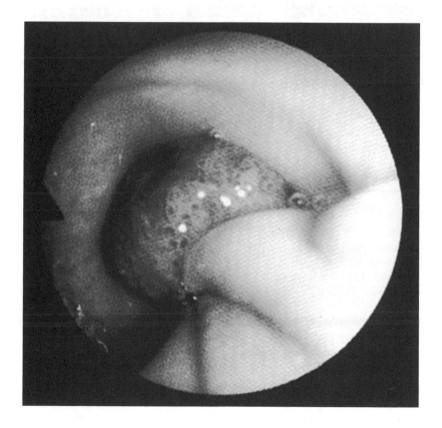

a. In 1 year
b. In 3 years
c. In 10 years
d. Repeat colonoscopy is not necessary

236. A 40-year-old male with long-standing alcohol abuse complains 6f abdominal swelling, which has been progressive over several months. He has a history of gastrointestinal bleeding. On physical exam, there are spider angiomas and palmar erythema. Abdominal collateral vessels are seen around the umbilicus. There is shifting dullness, and bulging flanks are noted. Which of the following is an important first step in the patient's evaluation?

a. Diagnostic paracentesis
b. UGI series
c. Ethanol level
d. CT scan

237. A 42-year-old man presents for the evaluation of splenomegaly, which was incidentally discovered on physical exam. You note mild abdominal distension with shifting dullness and perform diagnostic abdominal paracentesis. The fluid is straw-colored, nonbloody, and contains 320 white blood cells per μL, 68% of which are lymphocytes. The peritoneal fluid albumin level is 1.3 g/dL; the serum albumin level is 3.8 g/dL. Which of the following is the most likely diagnosis?

a. Portal hypertension
b. Pancreatitis
c. Tuberculous peritonitis
d. Hepatoma

238. A 63-year-old woman with cirrhosis due to chronic hepatitis C is hospitalized because of confusion. She has guaiac-positive stools and a low-grade fever. She has received lorazepam for sleep disturbance. On physical exam, the patient is confused. She has no meningeal signs and no focal neurologic findings. There is hyperreflexia and a nonrhythmic flapping tremor of the wrist. Which of the following is the most likely explanation for this patient's mental status change?

a. Tuberculosis meningitis
b. Subdural hematoma
c. Alcohol withdrawal seizure
d. Hepatic encephalopathy

239. A 50-year-old black male with a history of alcohol and tobacco abuse has complained of difficulty swallowing solid food for the past 2 months. More recently, swallowing fluids has also become a problem. He has noted black, tarry stools on occasion. The patient has lost 10 lb. Which of the following statements is correct?

a. The patient's prognosis is good
b. Barium contrast study is indicated
c. The most likely diagnosis is peptic ulcer disease
d. The patient has achalasia

240. A 34-year-old male presents with substernal discomfort. The symptoms are worse after meals, particularly a heavy evening meal, and are sometimes associated with hot/sour fluid in the back of the throat and nocturnal awakening. The patient denies difficulty swallowing, pain on swallowing, or weight loss. The symptoms have been present for 6 weeks; the patient has gained 20 lb in the past 2 years. Which of the following is the most appropriate initial approach?

a. A therapeutic trial of ranitidine
b. Exercise test with thallium imaging
c. Esophagogastroduodenoscopy
d. CT scan of the chest

241. A 48-year-old woman presents with a change in bowel habits and 10-lb weight loss over the past 2 months despite preservation of appetite. She notices increased abdominal gas, particularly after fatty meals. The stools are malodorous and occur 2 to 3 times per day; no rectal bleeding is noticed. The symptoms are less prominent when the patient follows a clear liquid diet. Which of the following is the most likely histological abnormality associated with this patient's symptoms?

a. Signet ring cells on gastric biopsy
b. Mucosal inflammation and crypt abscesses on sigmoidoscopy
c. Villous atrophy and increased lymphocytes in the lamina propria on small bowel biopsy
d. Small, curved gram-negative bacteria in areas of intestinal metaplasia on gastric biopsy

242. A nursing student has just completed her hepatitis B vaccine series. On reviewing her laboratory studies (assuming she has no prior exposure to hepatitis B), you should expect which of the following?

a. Positive test for hepatitis B surface antigen
b. Antibody against hepatitis B surface antigen (anti-HBs) alone
c. Antibody against hepatitis core antigen (anti-HBc)
d. Antibody against both surface and core antigen
e. Antibody against hepatitis E antigen

243. A 19-year-old woman is brought in by her mother because of chronic diarrhea. The young woman notes several nonbloody unformed stools a day. She has lost 5 lb of weight but is working out daily at a gym. She denies fever, chills, or perianal disease. Stool studies are negative for white cells or occult blood. Stool osmolarity is 300 mosm/L. The stool sodium is 35 and stool potassium is 40 meq/L. Which of the following is the most likely diagnosis?

a. Crohn's disease
b. Celiac sprue
c. Hyperthyroidism
d. Laxative abuse

244. A 40-year-old male has a history of three duodenal ulcers with prompt recurrence. Symptoms have been associated with severe diarrhea. One of the ulcers occurred close to the jejunum. Serum gastrin levels have been above 400 pg/mL (normal is 40 to 200 pg/mL). Which of the following is the most useful test in this patient?

a. Colonoscopy
b. Endoscopic retrograde cholangiogram
c. CT scan of abdomen
d. Secretin injection test

245. A 40-year-old white male complains of weakness, weight loss, and abdominal pain. On examination, the patient has diffuse hyperpigmentation and a palpable liver edge. Polyarthritis of the wrists and hips is also noted. Fasting blood sugar is 185 mg/dL. Which of the following is the most likely diagnosis?

a. Insulin-dependent diabetes mellitus
b. Pancreatic carcinoma
c. Addison's disease
d. Hemochromatosis

246. A 32-year-old white woman complains of abdominal pain off and on since the age of 17. She notices abdominal bloating relieved by defecation as well as alternating diarrhea and constipation. She has no weight loss, GI bleeding, or nocturnal diarrhea. On examination, she has slight LLQ tenderness and gaseous abdominal distension. Laboratory studies, including CBC, are normal. Which of the following is the most appropriate initial approach?

a. Recommend increased dietary fiber, prn antispasmodics, and follow-up exam in 2 months
b. Refer to gastroenterologist for colonoscopy
c. Obtain antiendomysial antibodies
d. Order UGI series with small bowel follow-through

247. A 55-year-old white woman has had recurrent episodes of alcohol-induced pancreatitis. Despite abstinence, the patient develops postprandial abdominal pain, bloating, weight loss despite good appetite, and bulky, foul-smelling stools. KUB shows pancreatic calcifications. In this patient, you should expect to find which of the following?

a. Diabetes mellitus
b. Malabsorption of fat-soluble vitamins D and K
c. Guaiac-positive stool
d. Courvoisier's sign

248. A 34-year-old white woman is treated for a UTI with amoxicillin. Initially she improves, but 5 days after beginning treatment, she develops recurrent fever, abdominal bloating, and diarrhea with six to eight loose stools per day. You suspect antibiotic-associated colitis. Which of the following is the best diagnostic test to confirm your diagnosis?

a.   Identification of *Clostridium difficile* toxin in the stool
b.   Isolation of *C. difficile* in a stool culture
c.   Stool positive for white blood cells
d.   Detection of IgG antibodies against *C. difficile* in the serum

249. A 27-year-old injection drug user presents with low-grade fever of 10 days duration and anorexia. Previous liver enzymes and HIV serology were normal. Physical exam is normal except for mild right upper quadrant tenderness. Liver enzymes at this time reveal ALT of 362 U/L (normal <40), AST 266 U/L (normal <40), bilirubin 1.2 mg/dL (normal), and alkaline phosphatase normal. Hepatitis C antibody is positive and HBc viral RNA is markedly elevated. Hepatitis B surface antigen is negative. Which of the following is the likely course of this illness?

a.   90% of patients resolve infection without lab abnormalities or clinical sequelae
b.   10 to 20% of patients resolve infection without detectable HCV RNA and normal liver function
c.   High likelihood of the development of cirrhosis
d.   Death within the next 6 months from progressive heptic failure

250. A 72-year-old woman notices progressive dysphagia to solids and liquids. There is no history of alcohol or tobacco use, and the patient takes no medications. She denies heartburn, but occasionally notices the regurgitation of undigested food from meals eaten several hours before. Her barium swallow is shown. Which of the following is the cause of this condition?

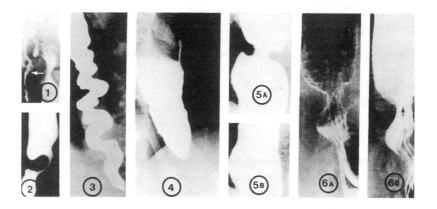

a. Growth of malignant squamous cells into the muscularis mucosa
b. Scarring due to silent gastroesophageal reflux
c. Spasm of the lower esophageal sphincter
d. Loss of intramural neurons in the esophagus

251. A 37-year-old woman presents for evaluation of abnormal liver chemistries. She has long-standing obesity (current BMI 38) and has previously taken anorectic medications but not for the past several years. She takes no other medications and has not used parenteral drugs or had high-risk sexual exposure. On exam her liver span is 13 cm, but she has no spider angiomata or splenomegaly. Several sets of liver enzymes have shown transaminases two to three times normal. Bilirubin and alkaline phosphatase are normal. Hepatitis B surface antigen and hepatitis C antibody are normal, as are serum iron and total iron-binding capacity. Which of the following is the likely pathology on liver biopsy?

a. Macrovesicular fatty liver
b. Microvesicular fatty liver
c. Portal triaditis with piecemeal necrosis
d. Cirrhosis

DIRECTIONS: Each group of questions below consists of lettered options followed by a set of numbered items. For each numbered item, select the **one** lettered option with which it is **most** closely associated. Each lettered option may be used once, more than once, or not at all.

Questions 252–254

Match the patient described with the most likely diagnosis.

a. Acute diverticulitis
b. Acute pancreatitis
c. Acute cholecystitis
d. Intestinal obstruction
e. Irritable bowel syndrome
f. Mesenteric ischemia

252. A 45-year-old moderately obese white woman presents after four episodes of severe epigastric and right upper quadrant pain, each episode lasting 30 to 60 min and accompanied by nausea and vomiting. Her most recent episode was very severe, with the pain radiating to the inferior angle of the scapula.

253. A 78-year-old white man presents with a 3-day history of gradually worsening left lower quadrant pain. He denies rectal bleeding or weight loss but has noticed mild constipation in association with the pain. He has a temperature of 100.2°F, moderate left lower quadrant tenderness without evidence of peritoneal inflammation, and a white count of 14,200.

254. A 68-year-old woman who has had a previous open cholecystectomy presents with an 8-h history of cramping periumbilical pain. Each episode of pain lasts 3 to 5 min and then abates. Over several hours she develops nausea, vomiting, and abdominal distension. She has been unable to pass stool or flatus for the past 4 hours.

Questions 255–256

Match the clinical description with the most likely disease process.

a. Primary biliary cirrhosis
b. Sclerosing cholangitis
c. Anaerobic liver abscess
d. Hepatoma
e. Hepatitis C
f. Hepatitis D
g. Hemochromatosis

255. A 40-year-old white female complains of pruritus. Physical examination reveals xanthelasma and mild splenomegaly. She has an elevated alkaline phosphatase, but her transaminases are normal. The antimitochondrial antibody test is positive.

256. A 30-year-old male with long-standing ulcerative colitis develops jaundice, pruritus, and right upper quadrant pain. Liver biopsy shows an inflammatory obliterative process affecting intrahepatic and extrahepatic bile ducts.

Questions 257–259

Match the clinical description with the most likely disease process.

a. Hemolysis secondary to G6PD deficiency
b. Pancreatic carcinoma
c. Acute viral hepatitis
d. Crigler-Najjar syndrome
e. Gilbert syndrome
f. Cirrhosis of liver

257. An African American male develops mild jaundice while being treated for a urinary tract infection. Urine bilirubin is negative. Serum bilirubin is 3 mg/dL, all unconjugated. Hemoglobin is 7 g/dL.

258. A 60-year-old male is noted to have mild jaundice and 15-lb weight loss. The patient has noted pruritus and pale, clay-colored stools. On exam the gallbladder is palpable. Alkaline phosphatase is very elevated.

259. A young woman complains of fatigue, change in skin color, and dark brown urine. She has right upper quadrant tenderness and ALT of 1035 U/L (normal is <40).

Questions 260–262

For each case scenario, select the most likely diagnosis.

a. Gastric ulcer
b. Aortoenteric fistula
c. Mallory-Weiss tear
d. Esophageal varices
e. Hereditary hemorrhagic telangiectasia (HHT)
f. Colon polyp
g. Adenocarcinoma of the colon

260. An 88-year-old white woman is taking naproxen for osteoarthritis. She has noticed mild epigastric discomfort for several weeks, but has continued the naproxen because of improvement in joint symptoms. She suddenly develops hematemesis and hypotension.

261. A 76-year-old white man presents with painless hematemesis and hypotension. He has no previous GI symptoms but did have resection of an abdominal aortic aneurysm 12 years previously. EGD shows no bleeding source in the stomach or duodenum.

262. A 23-year-old man develops iron-deficiency anemia and heme-positive stools. His weight is stable. A few telangiectasias are present on the lips. Abdominal exam is negative without hepatosplenomegaly.

Questions 263–265

For each case scenario, select the most likely diagnosis.
a. Ulcerative colitis
b. Crohn's disease
c. Ischemic colitis
d. Diverticulitis
e. Amebic colitis
f. Tuberculoma of the colon

263. A 35-year-old white man presents with diarrhea, weight loss, and RLQ pain. On exam, a tender mass is noted in the RLQ; the stool is guaiac-positive. Colonoscopy shows segmental areas of inflammation. Barium small bowel series shows nodular thickening of the terminal ileum.

264. A 75-year-old African American woman, previously healthy, presents with low-grade fever, diarrhea, and rectal bleeding. Colonoscopy shows continuous erythema from rectum to mid–transverse colon. The cecum is normal.

265. A 70-year-old white woman presents with LLQ abdominal pain, low-grade fever, and mild rectal bleeding. Examination shows LLQ tenderness. Unprepped sigmoidoscopy reveals segmental inflammation beginning in the distal sigmoid colon through the mid–descending colon. The rest of the exam is negative.

Questions 266–268

For each of the following case scenarios, select the most likely pathogen.

a. *Staphylococcus aureus*
b. *Shigella dysenteriae*
c. *Entamoeba histolytica*
d. *Giardia lamblia*
e. *Yersinia enterocolitica*
f. *Rotavirus*

266. A 21-year-old white male presents with 10-lb weight loss, abdominal bloating, and bulky, loose stools. He has no history of travel, but he does drink from a surface water source.

267. Two hours after ingesting potato salad at a picnic, a 50-year-old white woman develops severe nausea and vomiting. She has no diarrhea, fever, or chills. On exam, she appears hypovolemic, but the abdomen is benign.

268. A 30-year-old day care worker develops profuse bloody diarrhea, abdominal pain, and fever to 104°F. Exam reveals mild lower abdominal tenderness without rebound. WBC is 23,000 cells per μL. Several school-children have had a similar illness.

Gastroenterology

Answers

230. The answer is c. (*Kasper, pp 1895–1902.*) The Ranson criteria are used to determine prognosis in acute pancreatitis. Factors that adversely affect survival include age greater than 55 years, leukocytosis greater than 16,000/μm, glucose greater than 200 mg/dL, LDH greater than 400 IU, and AST greater than 250 IU/L. After the initial 48 h, a decrease in hematocrit, hypocalcemia, hypoxemia, an increase in BUN, and hypoalbuminemia are also poor prognostic findings. Hypotension with systolic BP less than 90 mmHg is also a poor prognostic sign; diastolic hypertension is not correlated with prognosis.

231. The answer is b. (*Kasper, pp 1751–1752.*) Localized epigastric burning pain relieved by eating requires evaluation for peptic ulcer disease. Upper gastrointestinal endoscopy provides the best sensitivity and specificity; barium swallow is less expensive, but is less accurate in defining mucosal disease. Patients with refractory or recurrent peptic ulcer disease should have serum gastrin levels measured to rule out gastrinoma. A positive antibody test for *H. pylori* would only indicate previous exposure.

232. The answer is c. (*Kasper, pp 1748–1751.*) *H. pylori* is present in 70% of patients who have a duodenal ulcer not associated with NSAID ingestion. In gastric ulcer disease, the incidence of *H. pylori* is 30 to 60%. *H. pylori* is more common in developing countries and in patients with low socioeconomic status, in particular those with unsanitary living conditions, which suggests that *H. pylori* is transmitted by fecal-oral or oral-oral routes. Before the discovery of *H. pylori,* most duodenal ulcers would reoccur.

233. The answer is c. (*Kasper, pp 1752–1757.*) Although acid suppression therapy leads to 80% healing rates after 4 weeks of treatment, acid reduction alone does not eradicate *H. pylori*. Three- or four-drug therapy, including bismuth or (most often) proton pump inhibitor, combined with two antibiotics effective against *H. pylori,* will be necessary to eradicate the organism. Longer duration of therapy (i.e., 14 days) leads to a greater healing rate.

This regimen will eradicate *H. pylori* in more than 90% of patients. Patients whose *H. pylori* has been eradicated have approximately only a 5% chance of ulcer recurrence (compared to 60 to 70% of patients not treated for *H. pylori*). Generally, follow-up tests to prove *H. pylori* eradication are not recommended in the usual patient who becomes asymptomatic. If the peptic ulcer should recur (again, this happens infrequently), either direct testing of a biopsy specimen or a test for urease activity in the stomach (i.e., the C13 breath test) is necessary, as the serological studies remain positive for many years.

234. The answer is a. *(Kasper, pp 1817–1821.)* Patients with jaundice should be characterized as having unconjugated (indirect reacting) or conjugated (direct) hyperbilirubinemia. Causes of unconjugated hyperbilirubinemia include hemolysis, ineffective erythropoiesis, or enzyme deficiencies (the commonest in adults being Gilbert's syndrome). The patient, however, has a conjugated hyperbilirubinemia, which almost always indicates significant liver dysfunction, either hepatocellular or cholestatic (obstructive); this patient's predominant elevation of alkaline phosphatase suggests a cholestatic pattern. Normal transaminases rule out disease-causing hepatocellular damage (such as viral or alcoholic hepatitis). Instead, a disease of bile ducts or a cause of impaired bile excretion should be considered. Ultrasound or CT scan will evaluate the patient for biliary or pancreatic cancer or stone disease versus intrahepatic cholestasis.

235. The answer is b. *(Kasper, pp 527–531.)* It is likely that most colon cancers start out as adenomatous polyps; this explains the rationale for using colonoscopy as a preventative test for colon cancer, despite the fact that proof is lacking. Larger polyps, sessile polyps, and those that contain villous elements are more likely to harbor malignancies. Patients who have had one adenomatous polyp removed have a 30 to 50% chance of developing another polyp, but the regrowth is slow (taking at leat 5 years to become clinically significant). Repeat colonoscopy is, therefore, recommended 3 years after the adenoma has been removed.

236. The answer is a. *(Kasper, pp 244–246, 1865–1867.)* Paracentesis is required to evaluate new-onset ascites. While cirrhosis and portal hypertension are most likely in this patient, complicating diseases such as tuberculous peritonitis and hepatoma are ruled out by analysis of ascitic fluid. An ultrasound or CT scan can be used to demonstrate ascitic fluid in equivocal cases.

237. The answer is a. (*Kasper, pp 244–246.*) A serum albumin minus ascitic fluid albumin greater than 1.1 suggests portal hypertension alone as a cause for ascites. Tuberculosis, pancreatitis, and malignancy would cause inflammation and increased capillary permeability, causing protein to leak into the ascitic fluid. This would result in a gradient between the serum and ascitic fluid of less than 1.1.

238. The answer is d. (*Kasper, pp 1867–1869.*) Hepatic encephalopathy presents as a change of consciousness, behavior, and neuromuscular function associated with liver disease. Hyperreflexia and asterixis (flapping tremor) are clinical manifestations of the disease process that result from toxins in the systemic circulation as a result of impaired hepatic clearance. Fever, gastrointestinal bleeding, and sedation are all potential precipitating factors in a patient with liver disease. Meningitis, subdural hematoma, and postictal state all occur in the alcoholic patient as well, and these may need to be distinguished from encephalopathy by additional tests such as lumbar puncture, CT scan, and EEG.

239. The answer is b. (*Kasper, pp 523–524.*) The most likely diagnosis in this patient is esophageal carcinoma. Dysphagia is progressive, first for solids and then liquids. There is blood in the stool and a history of weight loss. Alcohol use and cigarette smoking are risk factors. Prognosis is not good, as once there is trouble swallowing, there is significant esophageal narrowing and the disease is usually incurable. A barium contrast study should demonstrate an esophageal carcinoma with marked narrowing and an irregular, ragged mucosal pattern. Formerly squamous cell carcinoma accounted for 90% of esophageal cancer, but its incidence is decreasing. Now more than 50% are adenocarcinomas, most often associated with Barrett's esophagus. Achalasia should not cause guaiac-positive stools or progressive symptoms.

240. The answer is a. (*Kasper, pp 1742–1744.*) In the absence of alarm symptoms (such as dysphagia, odynophagia, weight loss, or gastrointestinal bleeding), a therapeutic trial of acid reduction therapy is reasonable. Mild to moderate GERD symptoms often respond to H_2 blockers. More severe disease, including erosive esophagitis, usually requires proton pump inhibitor therapy for 8 weeks before healing. If the patient has recurrent symptoms or has had symptomatic GERD for over 5 years, endoscopy may be indicated to rule out Barrett's esophagus (gastric metaplasia of the lower esophagus). Barrett's esophagus is a premalignant condition, and most patients receive surveillance EGD every 2 to 3 years, although evidence of mortality benefit from this approach is not available. In the absence of alarm symptoms, a therapeutic trial is generally favored over the more expensive invasive approach.

241. The answer is c. (*Kasper, pp 1768–1776.*) The patient's history suggests malabsorption. Weight loss despite increased appetite goes with either a hypermetabolic state (such as hyperthyroidism) or nutrient malabsorption. The gastrointestinal symptoms support the diagnosis of malabsorption. Patients may notice greasy, malodorous stools, increase in stool frequency, stools that are tenacious and difficult to flush, as well as changes in bowel habits according to the fat content of the diet. In the United States, celiac sprue (gluten-sensitive enteropathy) and chronic pancreatic insufficiency are the commonest causes of malabsorption. The histological pattern described in option c is associated with celiac sprue. IgA antiendomysial antibodies and antibodies against tissue glutaminase provide supporting evidence. Signet ring cells are seen with gastric cancer. This lesion can cause weight loss through anorexia or early satiety but would not cause malabsorption. The changes described in option b are associated with ulcerative colitis; since this disease affects only the colon, small bowel absorption would not be affected. *Helicobacter pylori* is not associated with malabsorption.

242. The answer is b. (*Kasper, pp 1832–1834.*) The current hepatitis B vaccine is genetically engineered to consist of hepatitis B surface antigen particles. Therefore, only antibody to surface antigen will be detected after vaccination. Since the patient has had no exposure to hepatitis B, she should be surface antigen–negative; surface antigen positivity means active disease, either acute or chronic. Patients who have recovered from hepatitis B have antibodies both to HBs and HBc.

243. The answer is d. (*Kasper, pp 224–231.*) Osmotic diarrhea is detected by finding an elevated osmolar gap in the stool. The formula for osmolar gap is:

$$\text{Stool osmolarity} - 2 \text{ (stool Na + stool K)}$$

An osmolar gap above 125 suggests that the diarrhea is caused by osmotically active particles in the stool. Laxative abuse, lactose intolerance, and the ingestion of sorbitol-containing foods are common causes of an osmotic diarrhea. This young woman was likely taking laxatives surreptitiously in an attempt to further lose weight. Inflammatory bowel disease is typically associated with white and red cells in the stool as well as systemic illness. Sprue may cause bulky, greasy, foul-smelling stools and weight loss despite increased caloric intake, although many cases are now diagnosed earlier with biochemical evidence of proxinal vitamin or nutrient malabsorption (hypocalcemia or iron or folate deficiency). The hyperdefecation of hyperthyroidism is due to a motility disturbance and would not widen the stool osmolar gap.

244. The answer is d. (*Kasper, pp 1758–1760.*) A young man with recurrent ulcer disease unresponsive to therapy should be evaluated for Zollinger-Ellison syndrome—gastrin-containing tumors that are usually in the pancreas. The patient's serum gastrin level is elevated, but not diagnostic for gastrinoma (>1000 pg/mL). A secretin injection induces marked increases in gastrin levels in all patients with gastrinoma. Once the diagnosis is made, CT scan or endoscopic ultrasound may help localize the tumor. Since these lesions arise from endocrine cells, they do not communicate with the pancreatic duct; ERCP would therefore not be helpful.

245. The answer is d. (*Kasper, pp 2298–2303.*) Hemochromatosis is a disorder of iron storage that results in deposition of iron in parenchymal cells. The liver is usually enlarged, and excessive skin pigmentation is present in 90% of symptomatic patients at the time of diagnosis. Diabetes occurs secondary to direct damage of the pancreas by iron deposition. Arthropathy develops in 25 to 50% of cases. Other diagnoses listed could not explain all the manifestations of this patient's disease process. Addison's disease can cause weight loss and hyperpigmentation but does not affect the liver or joints; it is associated with hypoglycemia rather than diabetes mellitus.

246. The answer is a. (*Kasper, pp 1789–1793.*) This patient meets the Rome II criteria for irritable bowel syndrome. The major criterion is abdominal pain relieved with defecation and associated with change in stool frequency or consistency. In addition, these patients often complain of difficult stool passage, a feeling of incomplete evacuation, and mucus in the stool. In this young patient with long-standing symptoms and no evidence of organic disease on physical and laboratory studies, no further evaluation is necessary. Irritable bowel syndrome is a motility disorder associated with altered sensitivity to abdominal pain and distention. It is the commonest cause of chronic GI symptoms and is three times more common in women than in men. Associated lactose intolerance may cause similar symptoms and should be considered in all cases. Patients older than 40 years with new symptoms, weight loss, or positive family history of colon cancer should have further workup, usually with colonoscopy.

247. The answer is a. (*Kasper, pp 1894–1895, 1902–1906.*) Chronic pancreatitis is due to pancreatic damage from recurrent attacks of acute pancreatitis. The classic triad is abdominal pain, malabsorption, and diabetes mellitus. Twenty-five percent of cases are idiopathic. Vitamins D and K are absorbed intact from the intestine without digestion by lipase and are therefore absorbed normally in pancreatic insufficiency. Forty percent of patients, however, develop B_{12} deficiency. Treatment of the malabsorption with pancreatic enzyme replacement will lead to weight gain, but the pain can be difficult to treat. Courvoisier's sign is a palpable, nontender gallbladder in a jaundiced patient. This finding suggests the presence of a malignancy, especially pancreatic cancer. Chronic pancreatitis per se does not produce guaiac-positive stools.

248. The answer is a. (*Kasper, pp 760–762.*) C. difficile is an important cause of diarrhea in patients who receive antibiotic therapy. C. difficile proliferates in the gastrointestinal tract when the normal enteric flora are altered by antibiotics. Commonly implicated antibiotics include ampicillin, penicillin, clindamycin, cephalosporins, and trimethoprim-sulfamethoxazole. The diarrhea is usually mild to moderate, but can occasionally be profound. Other clinical findings include pyrexia, abdominal pain, abdominal tenderness, leukocytosis, and serum electrolyte abnormalities. The diagnosis is made by demonstration at sigmoidoscopy of yellowish plaques (pseudomembranes) that cover the colonic mucosa or by detection of

C. difficile toxin in the stool. The pseudomembranes consist of a tenacious fibrinopurulent mucosal exudate that contains extruded leukocytes, mucin, and sloughed mucosa. Isolation of *C. difficile* from stool cultures is not very specific because of asymptomatic carriage, particularly in infants. Serological tests are not clinically useful for diagnosing this infection. Pseudomembranous colitis demands discontinuation of the offending antibiotic. Antibiotic therapy for moderate or severe disease includes oral vancomycin or metronidazole. Cholestyramine and colestipol are also used therapeutically to bind the diarrheogenic toxin.

249. The answer is b. (*Kasper, pp 1822–1838.*) This patient has acute hepatitis C. As is typical, the patient does not have jaundice. Symptomatic recovery from the acute illness is the rule, but most will have persistent transaminase elevation. All of these patients will remain positive for HCV RNA. Of the patients whose transaminases return to normal, a significant portion will remain positive for HCV and can develop progressive liver fibrosis despite the absence of symptoms. It is estimated that 20% of those who do not clear the hepatitis C virus will develop cirrhosis. Hepatitis B is more often severe in the acute phase, but only 10% of adults with acute hepatitis B will develop chronic disease. Although recovery from acute hepatitis A can be prolonged (up to 6 months), it does not cause chronic liver damage.

250. The answer is d. (*Kasper, pp 1741–1742.*) The barium swallow shows the dilated baglike proximal esophagus and tapered distal esophageal ring characteristic of achalasia. This is a motor disorder of the esophagus and classically produces dysphagia to both solids and liquids. Structural disorders such as cancer and stricture usually cause trouble swallowing solids as the first manifestation. In achalaia, manometry shows elevated pressure and poor relaxation of the lower esophageal sphincter. In classic achalasia the contractions of the esophagus are weak, although a variant called *vigorous achalasia* is associated with large-amplitude prolonged contractions. Medications (nitrates, calcium channel blockers, botox injections into the LES) or physical procedures (balloon dilatation or surgical myotomy) that decrease LES pressure are the recommended treatments.

251. The answer is a. (*Kasper, pp 1869–1871.*) This woman likely has nonalcoholic fatty liver (NAFL), which is associated with macrovesicular accumulation of fat in the liver. If hepatocellular necrosis is present, the condition is termed *nonalcoholic steatohepatitis* (NASH). This condition is histologically similar to alcoholic hepatitis, and increasing evidence suggests that it too is a precirrhotic condition. With the increasing incidence of obesity in Western societies, NASH may become the commonest cause of cirrhosis and end-stage liver disease. Microvesicular fat is seen in the acute life-threatening conditions of acute fatty liver of pregnancy and Reye's syndrome. Portal triaditis and piecemeal necrosis of cells in the hepatic lobule are associated with several disorders, including autoimmune and chronic viral hepatitis. Cirrhosis, characterized by bands of fibrous tissue, regenerating nodules, and disruption of the hepatic architecture, is the final common pathway of various chronic insults to the liver.

252–254. The answers are 252-c, 253-a, 254-d. (*Kasper, pp 1795–1797, 1803–1805, 1881–1887.*) Most gallstones are asymptomatic (about 15% of patients with incidentally discovered gallstones develop symptoms after 10 years). Symptoms of gallstones are usually caused by passage of a small stone down the cystic and common bile duct. While the stone is in the duct, it causes somewhat poorly localized visceral pain that is most often felt in the epigastrium or right upper quadrant. Usually the stone passes and the episode of biliary colic resolves after 30 minutes to 5 hours. If the stone becomes lodged in the cystic duct, acute cholecystitis develops. Acute inflammation causes distension and inflammation of the gallbladder, which then irritates the nerves of the parietal peritoneum. Then the pain becomes clearly localized to the right upper quadrant, becomes constant, and is associated with right upper quadrant tenderness and pain on inspiration (leading to Murphy's sign or respiratory arrest on palpation in the right upper quadrant).

Diverticula of the colon are also usually asymptomatic. More than 50% of patients over the age of 70 years will be shown to have diverticula by barium enema or colonoscopy. Symptoms of acute diverticulitis occur when microscopic perforation of the thin wall of the diverticular sac causes abdominal pain. Since diverticula are three times as common in the left colon as in the right, most acute diverticulitis is associated with left lower quadrant pain. Tenderness over the sigmoid colon is associated with mild peritoneal inflammation, low-grade fever, and leukocytosis. Evidence of generalized peritonitis is rare. Patients at this stage are usually managed with oral antibiotics; intravenous antibiotics are used if the patient suffers from vomiting or is severely ill. Antibiotics that cover usual colonic flora (gram-negative rods and anaerobes) will normally lead to resolution of diverticulitis. Diagnostic studies are generally deferred for several weeks for fear of worsening diverticulitis or causing perforation.

Acute intestinal obstruction is most often associated with adhesive bands from previous surgery. Hysterectomy and appendectomy are the most common preceding surgeries, although any operation associated with entry into the peritoneum can cause adhesions. The patient usually has the classic colicky pain associated with several pain-free minutes before the pain again builds up to maximum intensity. This kind of pain is much more commonly associated with intestinal obstruction than biliary or renal disease (so-called biliary and renal colic are often constant pains).

255–256. The answers are 255-a, 256-b. (*Kasper, pp 238–243, 1813–1816.*) Primary biliary cirrhosis usually occurs in women between the ages of 35 and 60. The earliest symptom is pruritus, often accompanied by fatigue. Serum alkaline phosphatase is elevated two- to fivefold, and a positive antimitochondrial antibody test greater than 1:40 is both sensitive and specific. Diverticulitis predisposes to liver abscess, particularly in the elderly patient. Obstructive jaundice that occurs in the setting of ulcerative colitis might be caused by gallstones or sclerosing cholangitis. Sclerosing cholangitis is a disorder characterized by a progressive inflammatory process of bile ducts. The diagnosis is usually made by demonstrating thickened ducts with narrow beaded lumina on cholangiography.

257–259. The answers are 257-a, 258-b, 259-c. (*Kasper, pp 238–243.*) The young African American male with mild jaundice has unconjugated hyperbilirubinemia and an anemia. This may be secondary to G6PD deficiency and an offending antibiotic (sulfonamide or trimethoprim-sulfamethoxazole). These patients are unable to maintain an adequate level of reduced glutathione in their red blood cells when an antibiotic or other toxin causes oxidative stress to the red cells. The 60-year-old male with jaundice has an obstructive process, as his pale stools suggest the lack of bilirubin in the stool. A high alkaline phosphatase also indicates that there is an obstructive jaundice. Pancreatic carcinoma would be the most likely cause of obstructive jaundice in this patient. The young woman's case is most consistent with acute hepatitis—very elevated hepatocellular enzymes and conjugated hyperbilirubinemia. Tenderness of the liver on palpation is common in acute hepatitis.

260–262. The answers are 260-a, 261-b, 262-e. *(Kasper, pp 235–238.)* Nonsteroidal anti-inflammatory drugs, even over-the-counter brands, are common causes of GI bleeding. Often, preceding symptoms are mild before the bleeding occurs. Cotreatment with misoprostol decreases GI bleeding but is quite expensive. Selective COX-2 inhibitors decrease the incidence of GI bleeding, but have recently been shown to increase cardiovascular events and to carry the same risk of renal dysfunction, edema, and blood pressure elevation as nonselective NSAIDs. Erosion of the proximal end of a woven aortic graft into the distal duodenum or proximal jejunum can occur many years after the initial surgery. Often, the patient will have a smaller herald bleed, which is then followed by catastrophic bleeding. A high index of suspicion is necessary, as surgery can be lifesaving.

Patients with HHT usually have low-grade GI blood loss without obvious hematemesis; frequent nosebleeds may occur. The physical finding of small matlike telangiectasias of the mouth, lips, and fingertips points to this autosomal dominant disease and may prevent unnecessary endoscopy.

263–265. The answers are 263-b, 264-a, 265-c. *(Kasper, pp 1776–1789.)* Crohn's disease can affect the entire GI tract from mouth to anus. Right lower quadrant pain, tenderness, and an inflammatory mass would suggest involvement of the terminal ileum. As opposed to ulcerative colitis (which is a mucosal disease), full-thickness involvement of the gut wall can lead to fistula and abscess formation. Skip lesions (i.e., segmental involvement) can also help distinguish Crohn's disease from UC; granuloma formation on biopsies would also support the diagnosis of Crohn's.

Although thought of as a disease of young adults, ulcerative colitis has a second peak of incidence in the 60- to 80-year age group and should be considered in the differential diagnosis of diarrhea at any age. Colonic involvement starts in the rectum and proceeds toward the cecum in a continuous fashion (i.e., no skip lesions). Inflammation is limited to the mucosa, so fistulas, abscesses, and granulomas are not seen.

Ischemic colitis also occurs in the older age group. The ischemia is usually confined to the mucosa, so perforation is unusual. Pain is a prominent complaint and may mimic acute diverticulitis. The finding of segmental inflammation in watershed areas in the vascular distribution of the colon is characteristic. Most patients improve without surgical intervention.

266–268. The answers are 266-d, 267-a, 268-b. *(Kasper, pp 225–227, 754–759.)* Giardiasis causes a subacute or chronic diarrhea with features of malabsorption. The protozoa plaster themselves to the small bowel mucosa and prevent intestinal absorption. Since the organisms are not invasive, white cells and RBCs are not seen in the stool. Travel history may suggest the diagnosis, but many cases are acquired from substandard drinking water supplies. A sensitive stool antigen test is now available.

Food-borne illness (food poisoning) is a very common cause of acute GI symptoms. The short incubation period (indicating a preformed toxin rather than bacterial proliferation in the body) as well as the prominent upper GI symptoms are characteristic of staphylococcal food poisoning. *Salmonella* food poisoning is also common, but has a longer incubation period, usually causes diarrhea, and may be associated with fever and guaiac-positive stools indicating tissue invasion. Numerous other bacterial agents can cause acute symptoms.

Shigella often causes severe diarrhea with high fever, leukocytosis, and clinical toxicity. Distal colon involvement can cause tenesmus. Only a few hundred organisms can cause clinical infection, so point source outbreaks are frequent.

Nephrology

Questions

DIRECTIONS: Each item below contains a question followed by suggested responses. Select the **one best** response to each question.

269. A 76-year-old male presents to the emergency room. He had influenza and now presents with diffuse muscle pain and weakness. His past medical history is remarkable for osteoarthritis, for which he takes ibuprofen. Physical examination reveals a blood pressure of 130/90 with no orthostatic change. The only other finding is diffuse muscle tenderness. Laboratory data includes:

BUN: 30 mg/dL
Creatinine: 6 mg/dL
K: 6.0 meq/L
Uric acid: 18 mg/dL
Ca: 6.5 mg/dL
PO_4: 7.5 mg/dL
CPK: 28,000 IU/L
Urine output: 40 mL/h

Which of the following is the most likely diagnosis?

a. Nonsteroidal anti-inflammatory drug-induced acute renal failure (ARF)
b. Volume depletion
c. Rhabdomyolysis-induced ARF
d. Urinary tract obstruction

270. A 73-year-old male undergoes abdominal aortic aneurysm repair. Postoperatively, his blood pressure is 110/70, abdominal aortic heart rate is 110, surgical wound is clean, and a Foley catheter is in place. His urine output drops to 40 cc/h, and creatinine rises from 1.5 to 2.2 mg/dL. Which of the following diagnostic tests is more useful for this patient?

a. Urine sodium
b. Urinalysis
c. Renal ultrasound
d. Urine uric acid–urine creatinine ratio

271. An 18-year-old male with a history of intravenous drug abuse develops status epilepticus. His CPK rises to 30,000 IU/L, his urine output drops to 20 mL/h, and his creatinine rises to 5.6 mg/dL. Which of the following is the best initial therapy for rhabdomyolysis-induced acute renal failure?

a. Mannitol
b. Dopamine
c. Natriuretic peptide
d. Alkaline diuresis

272. A 53-year-old male with septic shock develops acute renal failure with a serum creatinine of 6.4 mg/dL. Which of the following is a specific indication to initiate dialysis?

a. BUN rises to 75 mg/dL
b. Urine output falls to <10 mL/h
c. Pericardial friction rub develops
d. Hematocrit falls to <30%

273. A 68-year-old female with stable coronary artery disease undergoes angiography of the right lower extremity for peripheral vascular disease. The patient is on warfarin for recurrent deep vein thrombosis, aspirin, lisinopril, metoprolol, and atorvastatin. Preangiography, she received a course of dicloxacillin for cellulitis 1 week ago. Three weeks after angiography the patient is evaluated for general malaise. Physical examination reveals a petechial rash and livedo reticularis on both lower extremities. Laboratory evaluation reveals that her creatinine has risen from 1.5 to 3.7 mg/dL. Other laboratory abnormalities include an ESR of 96 mm/h, leukocytosis, eosinophiluria, and a reduced third component of complement (C_3). Urine sodium is 40 meq/L. Urinalysis reveals 2 to 4 eosinophils/HPF, 1+ protein, 10 to 20 WBC/HPF, and 5 to 10 RBC/HPF with no casts. Which of the following is the most likely diagnosis?

a. Prerenal azotemia
b. Radiocontrast-induced acute renal failure
c. Drug-induced acute interstitial nephritis
d. Atheroembolic renal failure

274. A 46-year-old male with HIV and severe penicillin allergy receiving zidovudine, indinavir, and stavudine presents with fever, nonproductive cough, and severe hypoxia. Chest x-ray reveals diffuse increased interstitial markings and a possible lobar consolidation in the left lower lobe. After appropriate evaluation, the patient receives levofloxacin, trimethoprim-sulfamethoxazole, and acyclovir. Initial serum creatinine is 1.6 mg/dL. On day 4, it has risen to 3.8 mg/dL and a normal serum potassium has risen to 7.1 mg/dL. Urinalysis reveals no casts, 10 to 20 WBC/HPF, and rare RBCs. Which drug is the most likely cause of renal failure?

a. Levofloxacin
b. Trimethoprim-sulfamethoxazole
c. Acyclovir
d. Indinavir

275. A 30-year-old male is brought to the emergency room from prison, where he works in the paint shop. He is barely arousable but has no focal abnormalities. He has no past medical history. CT scan of the head is normal. Urine toxicology screen is negative. Ethanol and acetaminophen are not detectable. Laboratory data is as follows:

Na: 138 meq/L
K: 4.2 meq/L
HCO_3: 5 meq/L
Cl: 104 meq/L
Creatinine: 1.0 mg/dL
BUN: 14 mg/dL
Ca: 10 mg/dL
Arterial blood gas on room air: Po_2 96, Pco_2 20, pH 7.02
Blood glucose: 90 mg/dL
Urinalysis: normal, without blood, protein, or crystals
Physical examination: blood pressure 100/60, with no orthostatic change

Which of the following is the most likely acid-base disorder?

a. Non-anion-gap metabolic acidosis
b. Respiratory acidosis
c. Anion-gap metabolic acidosis
d. Anion-gap metabolic acidosis plus respiratory alkalosis

276. A 20-year-old male presents acutely intoxicated. Blood pressure is 120/70. His laboratory values are as follows:

Na: 140 meq/L
K: 5.1 meq/L
Cl: 100 meq/L
HCO_3 15 meq/L
Creatinine 1.2 mg/dL
Blood ethanol: nondetectable
Blood glucose: 110 mg/dL
Arterial blood gases: Po_2 88, Pco_2 28, pH 7.28

Which of the following tests will provide the key to correct diagnosis?

a. Serum ketones
b. Serum lactate
c. Salicylate level
d. Measured plasma osmolality

277. A 70-year-old male is found lethargic at home with a blood pressure of 98/60 and a temperature of 98.6°F. In the emergency room, the following laboratory studies are obtained:

Na: 138 meq/L
K: 2.8 meq/L
HCO_3: 10 meq/L
Cl: 117 meq/L
BUN: 20 mg/dL
Creatinine: 1.0 mg/dL
Arterial blood gases: PO_2 80, PCO_2 25, pH 7.29
Urine pH: 4.5

Which of the following is the most likely acid-base disorder?
a. Non-anion-gap metabolic acidosis
b. Respiratory acidosis
c. Anion-gap metabolic acidosis
d. Non-anion-gap metabolic acidosis and respiratory alkalosis

278. A 17-year-old male is brought to the emergency room with confusion and incoordination. Laboratory values are as follows:

Na: 135 meq/L
K: 2.7 meq/L
HCO_3: 15 meq/L
Cl: 110 meq/L
Arterial blood gases: PO_2 92, PCO_2 25, pH 7.25
Urine: pH 7.5, glucose—negative
Ca: 9.7 mg/dL
PO_4: 4.0 mg/dL

Which of the following is the most likely cause of the acid base disorder?
a. GI loss due to diarrhea
b. Proximal renal tubular acidosis
c. Disorder of the renin-angiotensin system
d. Distal renal tubular acidosis

279. A 68-year-old female is found at home hypotensive (blood pressure 80/60) and confused. She has the following laboratory results in the emergency room:

Na: 130 meq/L
K: 2.6 meq/L
Cl: 70 meq/L
HCO_3: 50 meq/L
BUN: 40 mg/dL
Creatinine: 1.7 mg/dL
Arterial blood gases: PO_2 61, PCO_2 47, pH 7.63

Which acid-base disorder is present?

a. Metabolic alkalosis
b. Respiratory acidosis
c. Metabolic alkalosis plus respiratory acidosis
d. Respiratory alkalosis

280. A 73-year-old female with arthritis presents with confusion. Neurologic examination is nonfocal, and CT of the head is normal. Laboratory data include:

Na: 140 meq/L
K: 3.0 meq/L
Cl: 107 meq/L
HCO_3 12 meq/L
Arterial blood gases: PO_2 62, PCO_2, 24, pH 7.40

.What is the acid base disturbance?

a. Respiratory alkalosis with metabolic compensation
b. Metabolic acidosis with respiratory compensation
c. Metabolic acidosis and respiratory alkalosis
d. No acid-base disorder

281. A 43-year-old female presents with hypertension, edema, hyperlipidemia, and a deep venous thrombosis in her left leg. Which of the following is not necessary to diagnose the nephrotic syndrome?

a. Edema
b. Hypertension
c. 24-h urine albumin >3 g
d. Hyperlipidemia

282. A 63-year-old male alcoholic with a 50-pack-year history of smoking presents to the emergency room with fatigue and confusion. Physical examination reveals a blood pressure of 110/70 with no orthostatic change. Heart, lung, and abdominal examination are normal and there is no pedal edema. Laboratory data is as follows:

Na: 110 meq/L
K: 3.7 meq/L
Cl: 82 meq/L
HCO_3: 20 meq/L
Glucose: 100 mg/dL
BUN: 5 mg/dL
Creatinine: 0.7 mg/dL
Urinalysis: normal

Which of the following is the most likely diagnosis?
a. Volume depletion
b. Inappropriate secretion of antidiuretic hormone
c. Polydipsia
d. Cirrhosis

283. A 65-year-old diabetic male with a creatinine of 1.6 was started on an angiotensin-converting enzyme inhibitor for hypertension and presents to the emergency room with weakness. His other medications include a statin for hypercholesterolemia, a beta blocker and spironolactone for congestive heart failure, insulin for diabetes, and aspirin. Laboratory examinations include:

K: 7.2 meq/L
Creatinine: 1.8
Glucose: 400 mg/dL
CPK: 400 IU/L

Which of the following is the most important cause of hyperkalemia in this patient?
a. Worsening renal function
b. Uncontrolled diabetes
c. Statin-induced rhabdomyolysis
d. Drug-induced defects in the renin-angiotensin-aldosterone system

284. A 27-year-old alcoholic presents with the following electrolytes: calcium 6.9 mg/dL, albumin 3.5 g/dL, magnesium 0.7 mg/dL, phosphorus 2.0 mg/dL. Which of the following is the most important cause of the hypocalcemia?

a. Poor dietary intake
b. Hypoalbuminemia
c. Decreased parathyroid hormone release due to hypomagnesemia
d. Decreased end organ response to parathyroid hormone due to hypomagnesemia

285. A 27-year-old female presents to the emergency room with a panic attack. Electrolytes include calcium of 10.5 mg/dL, albumin 4.0 g/dL, phosphorus 0.8 mg/dL, and magnesium of 1.0 mg/dL. Arterial blood gases include a pH of 7.56, P_{CO_2} 21 mmHg, P_{O_2} 99 mmHg. Which of the following is the most important cause of the hypophosphatemia?

a. Hypomagnesemia
b. Hyperparathyroidism
c. Respiratory alkalosis
d. Poor dietary intake

286. A diabetic male presents with hypertension and 24-h urine showing 200 mg of albumin. In a diabetic patient with microalbuminuria, which of the following is the appropriate drug for treatment of hypertension to prevent progression of renal failure?

a. Beta blocker
b. Thiazide diuretic
c. Angiotensin-converting enzyme inhibitor
d. Short-acting dihydropyridine calcium channel blocker for precise control (nifedipine)

287. A 29-year-old male with HIV, on indinavir, zidovudine, and stavudine, presents with severe edema and a serum creatinine of 2.0 mg/dL. He
has had bone pain for 5 years and takes large amounts of acetominophen
with codeine, aspirin, and ibuprofen. He is on prophylactic trimethoprim
sulfamethoxazole. Blood pressure is 170/110; urinalysis shows 4+ protein,
5 to 10 RBC, 0 WBC; 24-h urine protein is 6.2 g. Which of the following is
the most likely cause of his renal disease?

a. Indinavir toxicity
b. Analgesic nephropathy
c. Trimethoprim sulfamethoxazole–induced interstitial nephritis
d. Focal glomerulosclerosis

288. A 60-year-old male is brought in by ambulance and is unable to
speak. The EMS personnel tell you that a neighbor informed them he has
had a stroke in the past. There are no family members present. His serum
sodium is 118 meq/L. Which of the following is the most helpful first step
in the assessment of this patient's hyponatremia?

a. Order a chest X-ray
b. Place a Foley catheter to obtain urine sample
c. Determine extracellular fluid volume status
d. Order a head CT scan
e. Order a urine Na⁺ level

DIRECTIONS: Each group of questions below consists of lettered
options followed by a set of numbered items. For each numbered item,
select the **one** lettered option with which it is **most** closely associated. Each
lettered option may be used once, more than once, or not at all.

Questions 289–292

Match the clinical and microscopic presentation with the correct primary glomerular disease.

a. Minimal change disease
b. IgA nephropathy
c. Focal segmental sclerosis
d. Thin basement membrane disease
e. Membranous nephropathy
f. Membranoproliferative glomerulonephritis

289. A 28-year-old black male presents with hypertension, nephrotic syndrome, renal insufficiency, microhematuria, and sclerotic changes in juxtamedullary nephrons.

290. A 50-year-old white male presents with mild hypertension, nephrotic syndrome, microhematuria, venous thromboses (including renal vein thrombosis), and thickened glomerular basement membrane with subepithelial immunoglobulin deposition.

291. A 17-year-old white male presents with normal blood pressure, anasarca, severe nephrotic syndrome, normal light microscopy, and fusion of foot processes on electron microscopy.

292. A 19-year-old white male presents with hypertension, nephrotic syndrome, mild renal insufficiency, RBC casts in urine, depressed third component of complement (C_3), and dense deposits on electron microscopy.

Questions 293–296

Match the presentation with the systemic vasculitis.
a. Macroscopic polyarteritis nodosa
b. Wegener's granulomatosis
c. Goodpasture's syndrome
d. Churg-Strauss syndrome - Autoimmune vasc. PAN, pANCA, lungs stue asthma
e. Essential mixed cryoglobulinemia
f. Systemic lupus erythematosus

293. An elderly male presents with severe hypertension, abdominal pain, livedo reticularis, and mononeuritis multiplex.

294. A Hispanic female, age 26, presents with a malar rash, arthralgias of the hands, and edema.

295. An older male presents with sinopulmonary disease and rapidly progressive renal failure.

296. A 35-year-old male with a history of intravenous drug abuse presents with a purpuric rash on his legs, hypertension, and hematuria.

Questions 297–299

Match the type of stone with the clinical situation in which it occurs.

a. Calcium phosphate
b. Calcium oxalate
c. Cystine
d. Struvite
e. Uric acid
f. Xanthine

297. A 50-year-old man with arthritis is on urinalysis and has a low urine pH.

298. A 40-year-old paraplegic has chronically infected urine.

299. A 23-year-old has hexagonal urinary crystals (intractable stone disease beginning in childhood).

Nephrology

Answers

269. The answer is c. *(Kasper, pp 1069, 1646–1647.)* Rhabdomyolysis-induced ARF may follow influenza. It is characterized by a creatinine disproportionately elevated compared to BUN (usual BUN-creatinine ratio is 10), hyperkalemia, hyperphosphatemia, and hyperuricemia, all due to release of intracellular muscle products. The high phosphorus causes hypocalcemia. All nonsteroidal agents may cause decreased renal function. Usually this is due to decreased blood flow—less commonly, to drug-induced interstitial nephritis. The laboratory abnormalities discussed are not caused by decreased blood flow or by interstitial nephritis. However, stopping the ibuprofen in this patient would be prudent. The absence of orthostatic hypotension makes the diagnosis of volume depletion very unlikely. Nothing on history, physical examination, or electrolyte abnormalities suggests obstruction. However, in a 76-year-old man, considering occult obstruction is always appropriate.

270. The answer is b. *(Kasper, p 1649.)* Urinalysis would be the best test because it is likely to show muddy brown granular casts, diagnostic of acute tubular necrosis and consistent with rhabdomyolysis-induced ARF. In oliguric (less than 20 mL urine per hour) ARF, a urine sodium less than 10 meq/L suggests prerenal azotemia; a value greater than 20 meq/L suggests acute tubular necrosis. Urine sodium is not useful in nonoliguric ARF (greater than 20 mL urine per hour). Obstructive uropathy is unlikely with the multiple electrolyte disorders in this patient. However, renal ultrasound is an appropriate test in a 76-year-old male to be sure occult obstruction is not contributing to renal failure. Despite the high serum uric acid, acute urate nephropathy does not occur with rhabdomyolysis. Acute urate nephropathy may occur with chemotherapy of aggressive tumors (e.g., Burkitt's lymphoma) and is characterized by a urine uric acid–creatinine ratio greater than 1.

271. The answer is d. *(Kasper, p 1650.)* Rhabdomyolysis-induced ARF is partly due to tubular obstruction by myoglobin and partly due to nephrotoxicity of myoglobin. Diuresis may relieve obstruction, and alkalization of the urine with bicarbonate may decrease nephrotoxicity of myoglobin. Frequently used in the past, mannitol no longer has a role in ARF. Low-dose dopamine may increase renal blood flow, but does not improve ARF. Natriuretic peptide has many theoretical hemodynamic effects, but has not been proved to improve ARF.

272. The answer is c. *(Kasper, pp 1650–1652.)* Pericarditis in renal failure (acute or chronic) is an indication to initiate hemodialysis, because untreated uremic pericarditis may progress to pericardial tamponade. Other indications include encephalopathy, volume overload, and intractable hyperkalemia. There is no absolute BUN number to initiate dialysis, although 100 mg/dL has been suggested. No degree of oliguria is a specific indication for dialysis, although this situation must be closely watched for volume overload. Bone marrow depression, mainly due to reduced erythropoetin combined with mildly reduced red cell half-life, causes hematocrit to fall almost universally in renal failure (acute and chronic). This does not determine need for dialysis.

273. The answer is d. *(Kasper, p 1647.)* Atheroembolic renal failure is a poorly understood syndrome of subacute renal failure in patients with severe vascular disease who undergo angiography. For unknown reasons, warfarin appears to be a risk factor. Clinical features include the dermatologic findings in this patient, refractile plaques in the retinal arteries (Hollenhorst plaques), and digital cyanosis. Although atheroembolic renal failure was once felt to lead inevitably to end-stage renal disease, it is now recognized that a significant percentage of patients have some recovery of renal function. Volume depletion is not associated with the physical findings and diverse laboratory abnormalities seen in this patient. In addition, a urine sodium less than 10 meq/L would be expected if the patient is oliguric. Radiocontrast-induced acute renal failure occurs immediately after contrast studies and lacks the physical findings and diverse laboratory abnormalities seen in this patient. Dicloxacillin may cause drug-induced acute interstitial nephritis, which is characterized by fever, diffuse erythematous rash, white blood cell casts in the urine, and eosinophiluria.

274. The answer is b. *(Kasper, p 1645.)* In the elderly or in patients with renal insufficiency, full doses of trimethoprim-sulfamethonazole frequently cause drug-induced interstitial nephritis and hyperkalemia (due to inhibition of the sodium-potassium transport system in the distal nephron). Levofloxacin is a very rare cause of renal dysfunction. In the setting of volume depletion, acyclovir may cause acute renal failure secondary to intratubular obstruction from crystal deposition. Crystals are absent from the urine in this case. Indinavir may crystallize and cause either nephrolithiasis or renal failure due to tubular obstruction.

275. The answer is c. (*Kasper, pp 265–266.*) The pH is low, so the primary process is acidosis. The serum HCO_3 has decreased from 24 to 5 meq/L, so this is a metabolic acidosis. The PCO_2 is 20 mmHg, down from a normal 40 mmHg, a normal compensation (PCO_2 decreases by 1 to 1.5 mmHg for each 1-meq decrease in HCO_3). The normal anion gap ($Na - [Cl + HCO_3]$) is 8 to 12 meq/L; here it is 29 meq/L. Thus this is an anion-gap metabolic acidosis with appropriate respiratory compensation. A brief differential of anion-gap metabolic acidosis is as follows:

Diabetic ketoacidosis
Lactic acidosis
Alcoholic ketoacidosis
Toxic alcohol ingestion (methanol, ethylene glycol)
Salicylate intoxication
Renal failure

Non-anion-gap metabolic acidosis is excluded by the anion gap of 31. Respiratory acidosis is excluded by the low PCO_2. Anion-gap metabolic acidosis plus respiratory alkalosis is excluded because the PCO_2 of 20 mmHg is appropriate compensation, not true respiratory alkalosis.

276. The answer is d. (*Kasper, pp 266–267.*) Plasma osmolality is calculated as follows: $2 \times Na + BUN/2.8 + glucose/18 + blood\ ethanol/4.6$ (denominators are a function of molecular weight). Here the calculated osmolality is 288 mosm/L ($2 \times 138 + 14/2.8 + 90/18 + 0/4.6$). Assume a measured plasma osmolality of 320 mosm/L. The measured osmolality of 320 mosm/L minus the calculated osmolality of 288 mosm/L is 32 (normal is less than 10), consistent with a large osmolar gap, due either to methanol or ethylene glycol. In this case, methanol, used in paint thinners, is likely. Ethylene glycol, used in antifreeze, is frequently associated with hypocalcemia, renal failure, and crystalluria. Serum ketones should be checked, but diabetic ketoacidosis is unlikely with a blood sugar of 90 mg/dL, and alcoholic ketoacidosis rarely, if ever, causes acidosis of this severity. Serum lactate should be checked, but in an afebrile patient with normal blood pressure lactic acidosis is unlikely to be the primary cause. Elevated salicylate level causes mixed metabolic acidosis–respiratory alkalosis with a near normal pH in the adult. In an infant, severe metabolic acidosis may occur.

277. The answer is a. *(Kasper, pp 265, 267.)* With a pH of 7.29, the primary process is acidosis. The HCO_3 is low (10 meq/L) and the anion gap is normal at 11 meq/L, and the PCO_2 of 25 mmHg is appropriate respiratory compensation. Thus this is a non-anion-gap metabolic acidosis with appropriate respiratory compensation. A brief differential diagnosis is as follows:

GI HCO_3 loss below the ligament of Treitz
Renal HCO_3 (proximal renal tubular acidosis)
Defects of the renin-angiotensin-aldosterone axis
Early chronic renal failure

Respiratory acidosis is not consistent with PCO_2 of 25 mmHg. Anion-gap metabolic acidosis is not consistent with a normal anion gap. Non-anion-gap metabolic acidosis and respiratory alkalosis are not present because the PCO_2 represents normal compensation for acute acidosis.

278. The answer is d. *(Kasper, pp 263–265.)* The patient has a non-anion-gap metabolic acidosis. Urine pH should be low, and a high urine pH is diagnostic of renal tubular acidosis (RTA). Proximal RTA is associated with glycosuria, phosphaturia, and aminoaciduria (Fanconi's syndrome). Since the serum phosphorus is normal and glycosuria is absent, proximal RTA is unlikely. GI Loss of HCO_3 due to diarrhea would be associated with an acid urine (pH less than 6). Disorders of the renin-angiotensin-aldosterone system are associated with hyperkalemia, not hypokalemia.

279. The answer is a. *(Kasper, pp 267–269.)* The pH is high and the plasma HCO_3 is high, consistent with metabolic alkalosis. The respiratory compensation is limited by hypoxic drive. Usually when the PCO_2 rises to the high 40s or low 50s, hypoxic drive is stimulated to maintain a PO_2 greater than 60 mmHg as in the present case. A brief differential diagnosis of metabolic acidosis is as follows:

Low or normal blood pressure
Upper GI loss above the ligament of Treitz
Renal loss (e.g., due to diuretics)
Increased blood pressure

Primary aldosteronism
Cushing's disease or syndrome
Any mineralocorticoid excess
Miscellaneous
Bartter syndrome

Respiratory acidosis cannot be the primary abnormality with high pH. Metabolic alkalosis plus respiratory acidosis is excluded because the increased PCO_2 represents appropriate compensation, not a primary disorder. Respiratory alkalosis is impossible with high PCO_2.

280. The answer is c. (*Kasper, pp 265–266.*) A normal pH, a decreased HCO_3 (with an increased anion gap) and a decreased PCO_2 mean metabolic acidosis plus respiratory alkalosis. This is the classic acid-base disturbance associated with aspirin intoxication. Choices a and b are wrong because compensation never normalizes the pH—the stimulus to compensate would be gone. Choice d is wrong because, while the pH is normal, the HCO_3 and PCO_2 are abnormal.

281. The answer is b. (*Kasper, pp 1684–1685.*) While hypertension may occur in diseases causing the nephrotic syndrome, its presence is not necessary for the diagnosis of this syndrome. Renal loss and catabolism of albumin lead to hypoalbuminemia and edema. Increased hepatic synthesis of lipoproteins leads to markedly elevated lipid levels.

282. The answer is b. (*Kasper, pp 254–256.*) Inappropriate secretion of antidiuretic hormone is a diagnosis of exclusion, but a chest x-ray might reveal a lung mass. This syndrome may be idiopathic, associated with certain pulmonary and intracranial pathologies, due to endocrine disorders (e.g., hypothyroidism), or drug-induced (e.g., many psychotropic agents). Significant volume depletion is excluded by the absence of orthostatic hypotension. As one can excrete 20% of the glomerular filtration rate, one would have to ingest more than 20 L/day to become hyponatremic. Cirrhosis is unlikely in the absence of ascites and edema.

283. The answer is d. (*Kasper, pp 261–262.*) The syndrome of hyporeninemic hypoaldosteronism occurs in older diabetic patients, particularly males with congestive heart failure. The syndrome often presents when aggravating drugs are added. Beta blockers impair renin secretion; converting enzyme inhibitors decrease aldosterone levels; and spironolactone competes for the aldosterone receptor. Combined with diabetes and mild renal insufficiency, the result may be significant hyperkalemia. The moderate increase in creatinine is unlikely to cause severe hyperkalemia. The hypertonicity due to hyperglycemia could aggravate hyperkalemia, but a blood glucose of 400 mg/dL should not cause severe hyperkalemia. Statin drugs may cause muscle injury and rhabdomyolysis, but a CPK of 400 IU/L is a modest elevation and would not cause severe hyperkalemia.

284. The answer is d. *(Kasper, pp 2244–2245.)* The major effect of hypomagnesemia on parathyroid hormone is decreased end organ response, including bone resistance and reduced renal synthesis of $1,25(OH)_2D$. A less important effect is impaired hormone release. Hypoalbuminemia decreases the serum calcium by 0.8 mgCa/g albumin and is a minor factor. Due to parathyroid hormone, dietary intake is a less important factor.

285. The answer is c. *(Kasper, pp 2241–2243.)* Respiratory alkalosis is one of the commonest causes of hypophosphatemia; it is due to intracellular shifts. Hypomagnesemia alone would increase phosphorus by decreasing parathormone effect. Hyperparathyroidism can decrease phosphorus, but not to this degree; also, calcium is not elevated. Severe hypophosphatemia is seen with poor intake, but occurs during the refeeding stage with carbohydrate intake.

286. The answer is c. *(Kasper, pp 1710–1714.)* By a variety of mechanisms, angiotensin-converting enzyme inhibitors help to preserve renal function in this situation. Angiotensin receptor blockers or the combination are favored by some. Two caveats: be sure to monitor serum potassium, and, in the older patient with potential renal vascular disease, monitor serum creatinine after initiation of therapy. Although many diabetic patients receive beta blockers due to coronary disease, these are not first-line drugs for preventing progression of renal failure. Caution is necessary in using beta blockers, as they may blunt the symptoms and physiologic response to hypoglycemia. Because of low cost and proven efficacy, thiazide diuretics remain a good choice for the general population, but do not have a specific effect on progression of renal disease. Short-acting dihydropyridine calcium channel blockers (nifedipine) may increase the incidence of stroke and myocardial infarction, and have no role in the treatment of hypertension.

287. The answer is d. *(Kasper, p 1111.)* Although many glomerular lesions occur in association with HIV, focal sclerosis is by far the commonest etiology of this patient's syndrome. While focal sclerosis is more common in intravenous drug users than in homosexuals, the lesion is different than so-called heroin nephropathy. Indinavir toxicity may cause tubular obstruction by crystals and is a cause of renal stones, but does not cause nephrotic syndrome. Analgesic nephropathy is a frequently unrecognized cause of occult renal failure; this entity requires at least 10 years of analgesic use and rarely causes significant proteinuria. Trimethoprim-sulfamethoxazole may cause acute interstitial nephritis, but there is no fever, rash, WBC casts, or eosinophils in the urinalysis.

288. The answer is c. *(Kasper, pp 254–255.)* The first step in the clinical assessment if hyponatremia is a thorough history and physical exam, including the assessment of extracellular fluid status. Increased ECF in the setting of hyponatremia may be due to heart failure, hepatic cirrhosis, nephrotic syndrome, or renal insufficiency. A normal ECF in the same setting would indicate a disorder such as SIADH, whereas a decreased ECF would lead to a determination of urine Na^+ concentration to further determine whether the hyponatremia was due to extrarenal versus intrarenal sodium loss.

Determination of plasma osmolality is helpful in the setting of hyponatremia. Most patients with hyponatremia will present with a low plasma osmolality. A high plasma osmolality indicates disorders such as hyperglycemia and a normal plasma osmolality can indicate disorders such as hyperproteinemia and hyperlipidemia. In a clinical setting such as this, determination of ECF status as you are performing the physical exam (history would be limited due to patient's inability to communicate) would be most appropriate. You would not wait for the plasma osmolality before beginning assessment and development of an initial differential diagnosis. Helpful laboratory assessment in the face of hyponatremia includes plasma osmolality, urine osmolality, and urine K^+ and Na^+ concentration.

289–292. The answers are 289-c, 290-e, 291-a, 292-f. *(Kasper, pp 1685–1686.)* Focal segmental sclerosis is common in African Americans, frequently progresses to end-stage renal disease, and is relatively refractory to therapy. Membranous nephropathy is the commonest cause of idiopathic nephrotic syndrome in adults. One-third of cases improve spontaneously, one-third remain stable, and one-third progress to end-stage renal disease if untreated. The condition is fairly responsive to corticosteroid and cytotoxic therapy. Minimal change disease is commonest in children; hypertension or renal failure is rare, and generally the condition is responsive to corticosteroid therapy. Membranoproliferative glomerulonephritis is the rarest cause of idiopathic nephrotic syndrome in adults. Depressed C_3 is due to an autoantibody that is not pathogenic. Erratic clinical course and erratic response to therapy are typical.

293–296. The answers are 293-a, 294-f, 295-b, 296-e. *(Kasper, pp 1960–1967, 2004–2012.)* Macroscopic polyarteritis nodosa is a vasculitis of medium-sized blood vessels that causes renal artery aneurysms (severe hypertension), abdominal aneurysms (abdominal pain), and vascular damage to skin and peripheral nerves. Patients are most commonly older males and anyone who is hepatitis B surface antigen–positive. SLE has a predilection for young African American and Hispanic females and has protean manifestations, especially a malar rash, arthralgias of the hands, and renal involvement. It is associated with a positive ANA (rim pattern) and antibodies against double-stranded DNA. Wegener's granulomatosis is most common in older males with granulomatous inflammation of the upper respiratory tract and kidneys and is associated with a positive c-ANCA (antineutrophil cytoplasmic antibody) test. Associated with hepatitis C, essential mixed cryoglobulinemia most commonly affects the skin and kidneys. Treatment is aimed at the hepatitis with interferon and ribavirin.

297–299. The answers are 297-d, 298-c, 299-b. *(Kasper, pp 1710–1714.)* Uric acid stones are associated with low urine pH. Low urine pH (due to decreased NH_3 production by the kidney) is the commonest cause of radiolucent uric acid stones. Urate is underexcreted in an acid urine. Struvite stones are found in chronically infected urine. Especially with *Proteus* infections, urinary pH rises to 8, causing precipitation of $MgNH_4PO_4$ into staghorn calculi. Stones are opaque. Hexagonal urinary crystals are found in cystinuria, an uncommon hereditary disease that leads to urinary wasting of cystine, ornithine, lysine, and arginine (COLA). Cystine stones start early in life and if untreated progress to end-stage renal disease. Stones may be lucent or opaque. Regional enteritis of the small intestine leads to increased oxalate absorption and formation of calcium stones. Stones are radiopaque.

Hematology and Oncology

Questions

DIRECTIONS: Each item below contains a question followed by suggested responses. Select the **one best** response to each question.

300. A 55-year-old male is being evaluated for constipation. There is no history of prior gastrectomy or of upper GI symptoms. Hemoglobin is 10 g/dL, mean corpuscular volume (MCV) is 72 fL, serum iron is 4 μg/dL (normal is 50 to 150 μg/dL), iron-binding capacity is 450 μg/dL (normal is 250 to 370 μg/dL), saturation is 1% (normal is 20 to 45%), and ferritin is 10 μg/L (normal is 15 to 400 μg/L). Which of the following is the best next step in the evaluation of this patient's anemia?

a. Red blood cell folate
b. Iron absorption studies
c. Colonoscopy
d. Bone marrow examination

301. A 50-year-old woman complains of pain and swelling in her proximal interphalangeal joints, both wrists, and both knees. She complains of morning stiffness. She had a hysterectomy 10 years ago. Physical exam shows swelling and thickening of the PIP joints. Hemoglobin is 10.3 g/dL, MCV is 80 fL, serum iron is 8 μmol/L, iron-binding capacity is 200 μg/dL (normal is 250 to 370 μg/dL), and saturation is 10%. Which of the following is the most likely explanation for this woman's anemia?

a. Occult blood loss
b. Vitamin deficiency
c. Anemia of chronic disease
d. Sideroblastic anemia

302. A 35-year-old female who is recovering from *Mycoplasma* pneumonia develops increasing weakness. Her Hgb is 9.0 g/dL and her MCV is 110. Which of the following is the best test to determine whether the patient has a hemolytic anemia?

a. Serum bilirubin
b. Reticulocyte count and blood smear
c. *Mycoplasma* antigen
d. Serum LDH

303. A 70-year-old male complains of 2 months of low back pain and fatigue. He has developed fever with purulent sputum production. On physical exam, he has pain over several vertebrae and rales at the left base. Laboratory results are as follows:

Hemoglobin: 7 g/dL
MCV: 86 fL (normal 86 to 98)
WBC: 12,000/mL
BUN: 44 mg/dL
Creatinine: 3.2 mg/dL
Ca: 11.5 mg/dL
Chest x-ray: LLL infiltrate
Reticulocyte count: 1%

The definitive diagnosis is best made by which of the following?

a. 24-h urine protein
b. Greater than 10% plasma cells in bone marrow
c. Renal biopsy
d. Rouleaux formation on blood smear

304. A 64-year-old man complains of cough, increasing shortness of breath, and headache for the past 3 weeks. He has mild hypertension for which he takes hydrochlorthiazide; he has smoked one pack of cigarettes a day for 40 years. On exam you notice facial plethora and jugular venous distension to the angle of the jaw. He has prominent veins over the anterior chest and a firm to hard right supraclavicular lymph node. Cardiac exam is normal and lungs are without rales. What is the most likely cause of his condition?

a. Long-standing hypertension
b. Gastric carcinoma
c. Emphysema
d. Lung cancer
e. Nephrotic syndrome

305. A 28-year-old woman presents with a 3-day history of fever and confusion. She was previously healthy and is taking no medications. She has a temperature of 38°C and a blood pressure of 145/85. Splenomegaly is absent. Except for confusion the neurological exam is normal. Her laboratory studies reveal the following:

Hemoglobin: 8.7
Platelet count: 25,000
Peripheral smear: numerous fragmented RBCs, few platelets
LDH 562 (normal <180)
Creatinine: 2.7
Liver enzymes: normal
Prothrombin time/PTT/fibrinogen level: normal

Which of the following is the best treatment for her condition?

a. Platelet transfusion
b. Intravenous immunoglobulin
c. Plasma exchange
d. Intravenous cyclophosphamide

306. After undergoing surgical resection for carcinoma of the stomach, a 60-year-old male develops numbness in his feet. On exam, he has lost proprioception in the lower extremities and has a wide-based gait and positive Romberg sign. A peripheral blood smear shows macrocytosis and hypersegmented polymorphonuclear leukocytes. The neurologic dysfunction is secondary to a deficiency of which vitamin?

a. Folic acid
b. Thiamine
c. Vitamin K
d. Vitamin B_{12}

307. A 60-year-old asymptomatic man is found to have a leukocytosis on a preoperative CBC. Physical exam shows the spleen tip to be palpable 2 cm below the left costal margin. Rubbery, nontender lymph nodes up to 1.5 cm in size are present in the axillae and inguinal regions. Lab data includes the following:

Hgb: 13.3 g/dL (normal 14 to 18)
Leukocytes: 40,000/μL (normal 4,300 to 10,800)
Platelet count: 238,000 (normal 150,000 to 400,000)
Peripheral blood smear is shown in photo

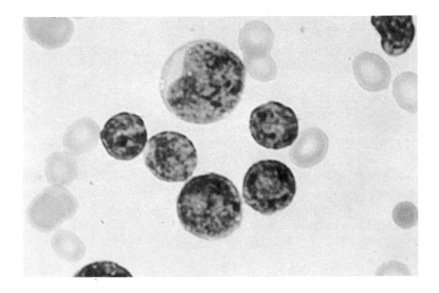

Which of the following is the most likely diagnosis?
a. Acute monocytic leukemia
b. Chronic myelogenous leukemia
c. Chronic lymphocytic leukemia
d. Tuberculosis

308. A 25-year-old woman complains of persistent bleeding for 5 days after a dental extraction. She has noticed easy bruisability since childhood, and was given a blood transfusion at age 17 because of prolonged bleeding after an apparently minor cut. She denies ecchymoses or bleeding into joints. Her father has noticed similar symptoms but has not sought medical care. Physical exam is normal except for mild oozing from the dental site. She does not have splenomegaly or enlarged lymph nodes. Her CBC is normal, with a platelet count of 230,000. Her prothrombin time is normal but the partial thromboplastin time is mildly prolonged. What is most appropriate way to control her bleeding?

a. Factor VIII concentrate
b. Fresh frozen plasma
c. Desmopressin (DDAVP)
d. Whole blood transfusion
e. Topical application of thrombin

309. A 67-year-old male presents with hemoptysis 1 week in duration. He has smoked 1½ packs of cigarettes per day for 50 years and has been unable to quit smoking despite nicotine replacement therapy and bupropion. He has mild COPD for which he uses an ipratropium inhaler. Chest x-ray reveals a 3-cm perihilar mass. Which of the following is the most likely cause of this patient's hemoptysis?

a. Adenocarcinoma of the lung
b. Squamous cell carcinoma of the lung
c. Bronchoalveolar cell carcinoma
d. Bronchial adenoma

310. A 38-year-old female presents with repeated episodes of sore throat. She is on no medications, does not use ethanol, and has no history of renal disease. Physical exam is normal. A CBC shows Hgb of 9.0 g/dL, MCV is 85 fL (normal), white blood cell count is 2,000/μL, and platelet count is 30,000/μL. Which of the following is the best approach to diagnosis?

a. Erythropoietin level
b. Serum B_{12}
c. Bone marrow biopsy
d. Liver spleen scan

311. A 50-year-old female complains of vague abdominal pain, constipation, and a sense of fullness in the lower abdomen. On physical exam the abdomen is nontender, but there is shifting dullness to percussion. Which of the following is the best next step in evaluation?

a. Abdominal ultrasound
b. Pelvic examination
c. CA 125 cancer antigen
d. Sigmoidoscopy

312. A 52-year-old man with cirrhosis due to chronic hepatitis C presents with increasing right upper quadrant pain, anorexia, and 15-lb weight loss. The patient is mildly icteric and has moderate ascites. A friction rub is heard over the liver. Abdominal paracentesis reveals blood-tinged fluid, and CT scan shows a 4-cm solid mass in the right lobe of the liver. Which of the following is the most important initial diagnostic study?

a. Serum α-fetoprotein level
b. Percutaneous liver biopsy
c. Measurement of hepatitis C viral RNA
d. Upper GI endoscopy
e. Positron emission tomography scans

313. A 40-year-old male complains of hematuria and an aching pain in his right flank. Laboratory data show normal BUN, creatinine, and electrolytes. Hemoglobin is elevated at 18 g/dL and serum calcium is 11 mg/dL. A solid renal mass is found by ultrasound. Which of the following is the most likely diagnosis?

a. Polycystic kidney disease
b. Renal carcinoma
c. Adrenal adenoma
d. Urolithiasis

314. A 64-year-old woman who is receiving chemotherapy for metastatic breast cancer has been treating mid-thoracic pain with acetaminophen. Over the past few days she has become weak and unsteady on her feet. On the day of admission she develops urinary incontinence. Physical exam reveals fist percussion tenderness over T8 and moderate symmetric muscle weakness in the legs. Anal sphincter tome is reduced. Which of the following diagnostic studies is most important to order?

a. Serum calcium
b. Bone scan
c. Plain radiographs of the thoracic spine
d. MRI scan of the spine

315. A 20-year-old male finds a mass in his scrotum. Which of the following is the most appropriate first step in evaluating this mass?

a. Palpation and transillumination
b. HCG and α-fetoprotein
c. Scrotal ultrasonography
d. Evaluation for inguinal adenopathy

316. A 65-year-old man presents with painless hematuria. He has a 45-year history of tobacco use. He denies fever, chills, and dysuria. General physical exam is unremarkable. On rectal exam, the prostate is small, nonnodular, and nontender. A urinalysis shows 100 red blood cells per high-power field. No white cells or protein are present. Three months previously, the patient had an abdominal ultrasound for right upper quadrant pain; on review, both kidneys were normal. Which of the following is the most useful diagnostic test at this time?

a. Urine culture and sensitivity
b. PSA
c. Renal biopsy
d. Cystoscopy

317. A patient complains of fatigue and night sweats associated with itching for 2 months. On physical exam, there is diffuse nontender lymphadenopathy, including small supraclavicular, epitrochlear, and scalene nodes. A chest x-ray shows hilar lymphadenopathy. Which of the following is the best next step in evaluation?

a. Excisional lymph node biopsy
b. Monospot test
c. Toxoplasmosis IgG
d. Serum angiotensin converting enzyme level

318. A 19-year-old woman presents for evaluation of a nontender left axillary lymph node. She is asymptomatic and denies weight loss or night sweats. Exam reveals three rubbery firm nontender nodes in the axilla, the largest 3 cm in diameter. No other lymphadenopathy is noted; the spleen is not enlarged. Lymph node biopsy, however, reveals mixed-cellularity Hodgkin's lymphoma. Liver function tests are normal. Which of the following is the best next step in evaluation?

a. CT scan of chest, abdomen, and pelvis
b. Liver biopsy
c. Staging laparotomy
d. Erythrocyte sedimentation rate

319. A 62-year-old African American man presents with fatigue, decreased urine stream, and low back pain. The physical examination shows a hard, nodular left prostatic lobe and percussion tenderness in the lumbar vertebral bodies and left seventh rib. Which of the following is the best next step in evaluation?

a. Bone scan
b. Biopsy of prostate
c. CT scan
d. Bone marrow biopsy

320. A 75-year-old man with a prior history of adenocarcinoma of the prostate treated with radical prostatectomy presents with pain in the left hip. The pain awakens him at night and has become increasingly severe over the previous 3 weeks. Plain radiographs show several osteoblastic lesions in the hip and sacrum, and the prostate-specific antigen level is 83 mcg/mL (normal 0 to 4). Which of the following is the treatment of choice?

a. Observation
b. Radiation therapy
c. Estrogen therapy
d. Gonadotropin-releasing hormone (GnRH) analogue
e. Chemotherapy

321. A 64-year-old male is hospitalized with a transient ischemic attack and is evaluated for carotid disease. Physical exam is normal. CBC on admission is normal. The patient is started on heparin. A repeat CBC 1 week later shows Hgb of 14 g/dL (normal is 13 to 18 g/dL), WBC of 9000/mL, and platelet count of 10,000/mL. Which of the following is the most appropriate course of action?

a. Obtain a bone marrow study
b. Obtain a liver-spleen scan
c. Suspect drug-induced thrombocytopenia
d. Begin corticosteroids for idiopathic thrombocytopenia purpura

322. A 73-year-old patient develops thrombocytopenia 5 days after coronary artery bypass surgery. Antibody titers against heparin/platelet factor 4 complexes are obtained, but, before the results are available, the patient develops thrombosis of the brachial artery. Which of the following is the best next step in management?

a. Begin warfarin
b. Begin thrombolytic therapy
c. Begin lepirudin or argatoban
d. Increase heparin dose

323. A patient with bacterial endocarditis develops thrombophlebitis while hospitalized. His course in the hospital is uncomplicated. On discharge he is treated with penicillin, rifampin, and warfarin. Therapeutic prothrombin levels are obtained on 15 mg/d of warfarin. After 2 weeks, the penicillin and rifampin are discontinued. Which of the following is the best next step in management of this patient?

a. Cautiously increase warfarin dosage
b. Continue warfarin at 15 mg/d for about 6 months
c. Reduce warfarin dosage
d. Stop warfarin therapy

324. A 65-year-old male with diabetes mellitus, bronzed skin, and cirrhosis of the liver is being treated for hemochromatosis previously confirmed by liver biopsy. The patient experiences increasing right upper quadrant pain, and his serum alkaline phosphatase is now elevated. There is a 15-lb weight loss. Which of the following is the best next step in management?

a. Increase frequency of phlebotomy for worsening hemochromatosis
b. Obtain CT scan to rule out hepatoma
c. Obtain hepatitis B serology
d. Obtain antimitochondrial antibody to rule out primary biliary cirrhosis

325. A 40-year-old cigarette smoker is found on routine physical exam to have a 1-cm white patch on his oral mucosa that does not rub off. There are no other lesions in the mouth. The patient has no risk factors for HIV infection. The lesion is nontender. Which of the following is the best next step in management?

a. Culture for *Candida albicans*
b. Follow lesion with annual physical exam
c. Refer to oral surgeon for biopsy of lesion
d. Reassure patient that this is a normal variant

326. A 37-year-old woman presents for evaluation of a self-discovered breast mass. There is no family history of breast cancer; she is otherwise healthy. Exam reveals a 1.5-cm area of firmness in the right upper outer quadrant. No skin changes are noted. You attempt to aspirate the mass, but no fluid is obtained; a mammogram is ordered and is normal. Which of the following is the most appropriate next step in management?

a. Refer the patient for further evaluation to a surgeon or comprehensive breast radiologist
b. Reevaluate the patient in 6 months
c. Give oral contraceptives to decrease ovulation and help shrink the lesion
d. Reassure the patient

327. A 47-year-old woman complains of fatigue, weight loss, and itching after taking a hot shower. Physical exam shows plethoric facies and an enlarged spleen, which descends 6 cm below the left costal margin. Her white cell count is 17,000 with a normal differential, the platelet count is 560,000, and hemoglobin is 18.7. Liver enzymes and electrolytes are normal; the serum uric acid level is mildly elevated. The most likely underlying process is which of the following?

a. Myelodysplastic syndrome
b. Myeloproliferative syndrome
c. Paraneoplastic syndrome
d. Form of Cushing's syndrome

328. A 20-year-old black male presents to the emergency room complaining of diffuse bone pain and requesting narcotics for his sickle cell crisis. Which of the following physical exam features would suggest an alternative diagnosis to sickle cell anemia (hemoglobin SS)?

a. Scleral icterus
b. Systolic murmur
c. Splenomegaly
d. Ankle ulcers

329. A 30-year-old black man plans a trip to India and is advised to take prophylaxis for malaria. Three days after beginning treatment, he develops dark urine, pallor, fatigue, and jaundice. Hematocrit is 30% (it had been 43%) and reticulocyte count is 7%. He stops taking the medication. Treatment should consist of which of the following?

a. Splenectomy
b. Administration of methylene blue
c. Administration of vitamin E
d. Exchange transfusions
e. No additional treatment is required

330. A 58-year-old Scandinavian male presents with shortness of breath and is found to have anemia. Peripheral blood smear shows macrocytosis and hypersegmented polyps. The patient also has postural hypotension. Skin shows both vitiligo and hyperpigmentation. Romberg sign is positive. Serum sodium is 120 meq/L (normal is 136 to 145 meq/L) and potassium is 5.2 meq/L (normal is 3.5 to 5.0 meq/L). Urinary sodium is increased. Which of the following is correct?

a. The patient's symptoms will be explained on the basis of folate deficiency
b. Only 50% of such patients will have parietal cell antibody
c. The patient is likely to have low levels of vitamin B_{12} and high levels of intrinsic factor
d. The patient is likely to have low levels of vitamin B_{12} and decreased secretion of intrinsic factor

331. A 78-year-old man complains of increasing fatigue and bone pain, especially around the knees and ankles. He has a long-standing anemia with a hemoglobin of 9 to 10 g/dL and MCV of 102. He had not responded to therapeutic trials of iron and vitamin B_{12}, but had been symptomatically stable until the past month. Examination reveals pallor and spleen tip just palpable at the left costal margin. CBC reveals hemoglobin of 8.2 g/dL, but for the first time his platelet count is low (15,000); the white blood cell count is 14,000. What is the likely cause of his worsening anemia?

a. Folic acid deficiency
b. Acute myeloid leukemia
c. Myelofibrosis
d. Tuberculosis
e. Viral infection

332. A 70-year-old intensive care unit patient complains of fever and shaking chills. The patient develops hypotension, and blood cultures are positive for gram-negative bacilli. The patient begins bleeding from venipuncture sites and around his Foley catheter. Laboratory studies are as follows:

Hct: 38%
WBC: 15,000/µL
Platelet count: 40,000/µL (normal 130,000 to 400,000)
Peripheral blood smear: fragmented RBCs
PT: elevated
PTT: elevated
Plasma fibrinogen: 70 mg/dL (normal 200 to 400)

Which of the following is the best course of therapy in this patient?
a. Begin heparin
b. Treat underlying disease
c. Begin plasmapheresis
d. Give vitamin K
e. Begin red blood cell transfusion

333. A 30-year-old female with Graves' disease has been started on propylthiouracil. She complains of low-grade fever, chills, and sore throat. Which of the following is the most important initial step in evaluating this patient's fever?
a. Serum TSH
b. Serum T₃
c. CBC
d. Chest x-ray
e. Blood cultures

334. A 54-year-old alcoholic woman presents with upper gastrointestinal bleeding and receives 4 units of packed red blood cells and 8 units of fresh frozen plasma. The bleeding stabilizes, but two days later the patient develops respiratory distress and hypoxemia. A chest X-ray shows bilateral infiltrates consistent with pulmonary edema. Which of the following is the likely cause of her respiratory symptoms?

a. Aspiration pneumonia
b. Pulmonary emboli
c. Transfusion reaction
d. *Pneumocystis carinii* pneumonia

335. A 64-year-old African American man presents for evaluation of a painless "lump" in the left thigh. He first noticed the abnormality about 1 month previously and thinks it has increased in size; there is no prior history of trauma. On exam, you find a 5-cm soft tissue mass, firm to hard in consistency, in the soft tissue above the knee. There is no tenderness or erythema; the mass is deep to the subcutaneous tissue and appears fixed to the underlying musculature. Inguinal lymph nodes are normal. Which of the following is the most appropriate management of this patient?

a. Reexamine the lesion in 3 months, as it is probably a lipoma
b. Obtain a bone scan
c. Treat with cephalexin 500 mg po qid for presumed abscess
d. Refer the patient for surgical biopsy

DIRECTIONS: Each group of questions below consists of lettered options followed by a set of numbered items. For each numbered item, select the **one** lettered option with which it is **most** closely associated. Each lettered option may be used once, more than once, or not at all.

Questions 336–338

Match the chemotherapeutic agent with the anticipated response.

a. Better than 50% chance that the lesion will be cured
b. Prolongation of survival
c. Palliation
d. Little or no response

336. A 25-year-old male has nonseminomatous testicular cancer and lung metastases.

337. A 56-year-old woman has malignant melanoma and lung metastases.

338. A 37-year-old woman has breast cancer and bone metastases.

Questions 339–341

Match the clinical description with the most likely diagnosis.
a. Sideroblastic anemia
b. Thalassemia
c. Iron-deficiency anemia
d. Anemia of renal disease
e. Anemia of chronic disease

339. An alcoholic patient being treated for tuberculosis has an increase in serum iron and transferrin saturation.

340. A 70-year-old Hispanic woman presents with weight loss, constipation, and heme-positive stools. She has a microcytic anemia with low serum iron and elevated iron-binding capacity.

341. A 52-year-old African American diabetic requires hemodialysis for end-stage renal disease. She has hemoglobin of 9, hematocrit of 27, and normal red cell indices. The iron and iron-binding capacity are normal.

Questions 342–344

Match the clinical description with the paraneoplastic syndrome most often associated with it.

a. Humoral hypercalcemia of malignancy
b. Hyponatremia due to inappropriate ADH secretion
c. Hypoglycemia due to IGF-2
d. Migratory thrombophlebitis due to procoagulant cytokines
e. Skin infiltration with T lymphocytes
f. Erythrocytosis due to erythropoietin

342. A 76-year-old woman presents with weight loss, depression, and anemia of chronic disease. CT of the abdomen reveals a 4-cm pancreatic mass.

343. A 48-year-old cigarette smoker complains of weight loss and hemoptysis. Chest x-ray shows a 4-cm hilar mass; transbronchial biopsy reveals squamous cell carcinoma.

344. A 58-year-old cigarette smoker develops a cough, weakness, and mental confusion. Chest CT shows a 2-cm perihilar density with hilar and mediastinal lymphadenopathy. Sputum cytology shows small, undifferentiated cells.

Hematology and Oncology

Answers

300. The answer is c. *(Kasper, pp 586–591.)* The patient has a microcytic anemia. A low serum iron, low ferritin, and high iron-binding capacity all suggest iron-deficiency anemia. Most iron-deficiency anemia is explained by blood loss. The patient's symptoms of constipation point to blood loss from the lower GI tract. Colonoscopy would be the highest-yield procedure. Barium enema misses 50% of polyps and a significant minority of colon cancers. Even patients without a history of GI symptoms who have no obvious explanation for their iron deficiency (such as menstrual blood loss or multiple prior pregnancies in women) should be studied for GI blood loss. Lead poisoning can cause a microcytic hypochromic anemia, but this would not be associated with the abnormal iron studies and low ferritin seen in this patient. Basophilic stippling or target cells seen on the peripheral blood smear would be important clues to the presence of lead poisoning. Folate deficiency presents as a megaloblastic anemia with macrocytosis (large, oval-shaped red cells) and hypersegmentation of the polymorphonuclear leukocytes.

301. The answer is c. *(Kasper, pp 591–592.)* Patients with chronic inflammatory or neoplastic disease often develop anemia of chronic disease. Cytokines produced by inflammation cause a block in the normal recirculation of iron from reticuloendothelial cells (which pick up the iron from senescent red blood cells) to the red cell precursors (normoblasts). In addition, IL-1 and interferon γ decrease the production of and the response to erythropoietin. This causes a drop in the serum iron concentration and a normocytic or mild microcytic anemia. The inflammatory reaction, however, also decreases the iron-binding capacity (as opposed to iron-deficiency anemia, where the iron-binding capacity is elevated), so the saturation is usually between 10 and 20%. The anemia is rarely severe (Hb rarely less than 8.5 g/dL). The hemoglobin and hematocrit will improve if the underlying process is treated. Diseases not associated with inflammation or neoplasia (i.e., congestive heart failure, diabetes, hypertension, etc.) do not cause anemia of chronic disease. Blood loss would generally cause a lower serum iron level, an elevated iron-binding capacity, and a lower iron saturation. The serum ferritin (low in iron deficiency, normal or high in anemia of chronic disease) will usually clarify this situation. Vitamin B_{12} and folate deficiencies are associated with a macrocytic anemia. Sideroblastic anemia can be either microcytic or macrocytic (occasionally with a dimorphic population of cells, some small and some large), but is not associated with a low iron level. In addition, this patient's history (which suggests an inflammatory polyarthritis) would not be consistent with sideroblastic anemia. The diagnosis of sideroblastic anemia is made by seeing ringed sideroblasts on bone marrow aspirate.

302. The answer is b. (*Kasper, pp 329–335, 607–616.*) An elevated reticulocyte count suggests active bone marrow response either to red blood cell loss (acute bleeding) or destruction (hemolysis). Many cases of hemolytic anemia can be diagnosed from changes on the peripheral blood smear. Large polychromatophilic cells suggest reticulocytes (which can be diagnosed with a reticulum stain). Microspherocytes suggest immune-mediated hemolysis. Fragmented cells suggest microvascular damage. This patient likely has immune-mediated hemolysis due to her *Mycoplasma* infection. This is usually associated with IgM antibodies, which react better at temperatures less than 37°C (and thus are called *cold-reacting antibodies*). The cold agglutinins associated with *Mycoplasma* typically react with anti-I cells. Those seen in infectious mononucleosis typically react with anti-I cells. Although the serum bilirubin and LDH are often elevated in hemolysis, they are less specific, and tests would usually be performed after the reticulocyte count and peripheral blood smear. The *Mycoplasma* antigen test would confirm recent infection with *M. pneumoniae* but would not specifically explain the cause of the anemia.

303. The answer is b. (*Kasper, pp 656–661.*) Multiple myeloma would best explain this patient's presentation. The onset of myeloma is often insidious. Pain caused by bone involvement, anemia, renal insufficiency, and bacterial pneumonia often follow. This patient presented with fatigue and bone pain, then developed bacterial pneumonia probably secondary to *Streptococcus pneumoniae*, an encapsulated organism for which antibody to the polysaccharide capsule is not adequately produced by the myeloma patient. There is also evidence for renal insufficiency. Hypercalcemia is frequently seen in patients with multiple myeloma and may be life-threatening. Definitive diagnosis of multiple myeloma is made by demonstrating greater than 10% plasma cells in the bone marrow. None of the other findings are specific enough for definitive diagnosis. Renal biopsy would not be helpful. About 75% of patients with myeloma will have a monoclonal M spike on serum protein electrophoresis, but about 25% will produce primarily Bence-Jones proteins, which, because of their small size, do not accumulate in the serum but are excreted in the urine. A urine protein electrophoresis will identify these patients. Less than 1% of patients with myeloma will present with a nonsecretory myeloma; the diagnosis can be made only with bone marrow biopsy. Renal biopsy might show monoclonal protein deposition in the kidney or intratubular casts but would not be the first diagnostic procedure. Rouleaux formation, although characteristic of myeloma, is neither sensitive nor specific.

304. The answer is d. *(Kasper, pp 575–576.)* This patient presents with the superior vena cava syndrome. Such patients have jugular venous distension but no other signs of right-sided heart failure. They have prominent facial (especially periorbital) puffiness and may complain of headache, dizziness, or lethargy. SVC syndrome is due to a malignant tumor 90% of the time. Lung cancer and lymphoma, both of which are often associated with bulky mediastinal lymphadenopathy, predominate. Gastric cancer often metastasizes to the supraclavicular nodes (most often on the left, the so-called Virchow's node) but does not usually affect the mediastinal nodes to this degree. Prompt diagnosis is necessary to prevent CNS complications or laryngeal edema. Sensitive tumors (lymphoma, small cell lung cancer) may be treated with chemotherapy, while most other cell types are treated with radiation therapy.

305. The answer is c. *(Kasper, pp 678–679, 1708.)* This patient has thrombotic thrombocytopenic purpura (TTP). TTP is an acute life-threatening disorder that is characterized by the pentad of microangiopathic hemolytic anemia, nonimmune thrombocytopenia, fever, renal insufficiency, and CNS involvement (confusion or multifocal encephalopathy). It may be triggered by endothelial damage and is associated with deficiency of a plasma protein (ADAMTS 13) that breaks down multimers of von Willebrand factor. Plasma exchange (with the infusion of fresh frozen plasma to provide the missing ADAMTS 13 protein) can be lifesaving. Disseminated intravascular coagulation associated with sepsis can resemble TTP, but the coagulation pathway is usually activated in DIC. In TTP the prothrombin time, PTT, and fibrinogen level are usually normal.

306. The answer is d. (*Kasper, pp 601–607.*) These neurologic deficits occur with vitamin B_{12} deficiency. This patient has a deficit of intrinsic factor after gastric surgery. Intrinsic factor is produced by gastric parietal cells and is a major factor in enhancing ileal absorption of B_{12}. Milder degrees of B_{12} malabsorption can occur after partial gastrectomy, probably due to decreased release of B_{12} from food. Folic acid deficiency causes identical megaloblastic changes in the blood but is not associated with the neurologic deficit (loss of proprioception) that occurs with B_{12} deficiency. Thiamine deficiency causes beriberi; Vitamin K deficiency causes a coagulopathy associated with ecchymoses and prolongation of prothrombin time. These vitamins do not depend on gastric factors for their absorption.

307. The answer is c. (*Kasper, pp 641–652.*) Chronic lymphocytic leukemia is the most common of all leukemias, with incidence increasing with age. Patients are usually asymptomatic, but may complain of weakness, fatigue, or enlarged lymph nodes. The diagnosis is made by peripheral blood smear, as mature small lymphocytes constitute almost all the white blood cells seen. No other process produces a lymphocytosis of this morphology and magnitude. The leukemic cells in acute leukemia are immature blast cells that are easily distinguished from the normal-appearing mature lymphocytes of CLL. Both chronic myelogenous leukemia and the leukemoid reaction associated with illness such as TB are associated with increased numbers of a variety of cells of the myeloid series (mature polymorphonuclear leukocytes, metamyelocytes, myelocytes, etc.). The peripheral blood is said to resemble a dilute preparation of bone marrow. The presence of basophilia would suggest CML.

308. The answer is c. (*Kasper, pp 676–677.*) This woman's lifelong history of excessive bleeding suggests an inherited bleeding problem, as does the positive family history. The prolonged PTT indicates a deficiency of either factor VIII, IX, XI, or XII, but the commonest of these deficiencies (classic hemophilia A and Christmas disease, or hemophilia B) are vanishingly rare in women. Furthermore, the continued oozing from dental sites and the absence of ecchymoses or hemarthroses suggest a platelet function disorder. Von Willebrand's disease is an autosomal dominant condition that leads to both platelet and factor VIII dysfunction. Although factor VIII concentrates can be used for life-threatening bleeding in these patients, most will respond to desmopressin, which raises the von Willebrand factor level in the most common form (the so-called type 1 form) of this disease. Mild von Willebrand disease is fairly common (1 in 250 individuals).

309. The answer is b. *(Kasper, pp 506–516.)* Cigarette smokers have a 15- to 25-fold increased incidence of both squamous cell carcinoma and small cell undifferentiated carcinoma of the lung. Both of these neoplasms tend to be central (i.e., perihilar); the presence of obstructive lung disease increases the risk of lung cancer over and above the smoking history. Of the choices given, squamous cell carcinoma is the likeliest explanation for this patient's hemoptysis. Bronchoscopy would likely show the lesion and allow a tissue diagnosis to be made. Adenocarcinoma of the lung is the commonest lung cancer seen in nonsmokers, women, and younger patients. Its incidence is increased in smokers (probably twofold), but not to the degree seen with squamous cell carcinoma and small cell undifferentiated carcinoma. Adenocarcinoma is typically peripheral with pleural involvement (rather than the central involvement seen in this case). Bronchoalveolar cell carcinoma arises from alveolar epithelium, is typically peripheral, and may resemble a nonhealing pneumonia (it may even have air bronchograms like a pneumonia). Bronchial adenomas (carcinoid being the commonest type) are often central but are usually smaller and are less common than squamous cell carcinomas. Their incidence is not increased by cigarette smoking.

310. The answer is c. *(Kasper, pp 617–624.)* This patient has an unexplained pancytopenia. If all three elements (red blood cells, white blood cells, and platelets) are affected, the cause is usually in the bone marrow (although peripheral destruction from hypersplenism can occasionally cause pancytopenia). In this patient without a history of liver disease or palpable splenomegaly on physical examination, a bone marrow production problem is the most likely culprit. Although B_{12} deficiency can cause pancytopenia, usually a macrocytic anemia is the most prominent feature; a serum B_{12} level would be reasonable, but the most productive approach would be to examine the bone marrow. Leukemia can present without leukocytosis (so-called aleukemic leukemia), but the most likely diagnosis would be aplastic anemia. In the elderly patient, myelodysplastic syndrome (MDS) may present with pancytopenia.

311. The answer is b. *(Kasper, pp 553–556.)* The first step in this patient's evaluation is a pelvic exam to check for ovarian cancer. Pelvic fullness, vague discomfort, constipation, and early satiety are often the first symptoms of this disease. Ascites may be present on initial evaluation. Abdominal ultrasound would follow. The CA 125 cancer antigen supports the diagnosis of ovarian cancer, but it is not sensitive or specific. If the pelvic exam and ultrasound were negative, sigmoidoscopy might be indicated to evaluate the patient's constipation.

312. The answer is a. *(Kasper, pp 533–535.)* This patient has probably developed hepatocellular carcinoma as a complication of her macronodular cirrhosis. HCC is a feared complication of patients with cirrhosis due to hepatitis B, hepatitis C, and hemochromatosis (although it occurs with modestly increased frequency in patients with alcoholic cirrhosis as well). The incidence in high-risk patients is 3% per year. An α-fetoprotein (AFP) level greater than 500 mcg/L is suggestive, and greater than 1000 mcg/L virtually diagnostic, of this tumor. Most patients will die within 6 months if untreated; resection of the tumor is often difficult due to the underlying liver disease. Liver transplantation can be curative in selected patients.

313. The answer is b. *(Kasper, pp 541–542.)* Renal carcinoma is twice as common in men as women and tends to occur in the 50- to 70-year age group. Many patients present with a hematuria or flank pain, but the classic triad of hematuria, flank pain, and a palpable flank mass occurs in only 10 to 20% of patients. Paraneoplastic syndromes such as erythrocytosis, hypercalcemia, hepatic dysfunction, and fever of unknown origin are common. Surgery is the only potentially curable therapy; the results of treatment with chemotherapy or radiation therapy for nonresectable disease have been disappointing. Interferon α and interleukin 2 produce responses (but no cures) in 10 to 20% of patients. The prognosis for metastatic renal cell carcinoma is dismal.

314. The answer is d. *(Kasper, pp 577–579.)* Spinal cord compression is an oncologic emergency. Major neurological deficit is often irreversible and severely compromises the patient's remaining quality of life. Vertebral and then epidural involvement precede the neurological findings; the thoracic cord is involved 70% of the time. The patient is often given high-dose dexamethasone before being sent for the MRI. In the presence of neurological compromise, the definitive test (MRI) scan should be performed as quickly as possible. Multiple epidural metastases are noted in 25% of patients; their presence can affect treatment (e.g., the extent of radiation therapy fields). If no neurological abnormalities are present, most experts recommend plain radiographs of the painful vertebra as the initial diagnostic test.

315. The answer is a. (*Kasper, pp 550–553.*) The first step in evaluating a scrotal mass is to determine whether the mass is in the testis or outside it. Most solid masses arising from within the testis are malignant. Palpation of the scrotal mass and transillumination (holding a flashlight directly against the posterior wall of the scrotum) will distinguish testicular lesions from other masses within the scrotum, such as hydrocele. Ultrasonography will confirm a solid testicular mass. The tumor markers β-HCG and α-fetoprotein are not used in the initial evaluation of a scrotal mass, but will be important for staging when a solid mass suggestive of testicular carcinoma is found. β-HCG or AFP will be elevated in about 70% of patients with disseminated nonseminomatous testicular cancer. Seminomas are usually associated with normal tumor cell markers. Choriocarcinomas produce β-HCG. Endodermal sinus tumors or embryonal cell carcinomas are often associated with elevated AFP levels. The lymphatic drainage of the testis is into the periaortic nodes, not to the inguinal nodes. The periaortic nodes must be assessed radiographically, usually by CT scanning, if a testicular neoplasm is found.

316. The answer is d. (*Kasper, pp 250–251, 539–541.*) Unexplained gross hematuria requires evaluation. Patients who have gross hematuria in association with clear-cut urinary tract infection are usually treated and followed with a repeat urinalysis to confirm clearing of the RBCs, but this patient has no symptoms of urinary tract infection. Although benign causes (prostatitis, renal stones) are most common, as many as 15% of patients with gross hematuria will have bladder cancer. Cigarette smoking increases the risk of bladder cancer two- to fourfold. Exposure to aniline dyes, chronic cyclophosphamide treatment, external beam radiation, and *Schistosoma* infection of the bladder are other risk factors. This patient should be referred to a urologist for cystoscopy to rule out transitional cell carcinoma of the bladder. If no lesion is found, CT scanning of the kidneys would be indicated despite the previous negative sonogram.

317. The answer is a. (*Kasper, pp 343–345.*) The long-term nature of these symptoms, the fact that the nodes are nontender, and their location (including scalene and supraclavicular) all suggest the likelihood of malignancy. Although infectious mononucleosis and toxoplasmosis can cause diffuse lymphadenopathy, these infections are usually associated with other evidence of infection such as pharyngitis, fever, and atypical lymphocytosis in the peripheral blood. It would be unusual for the lymphadenopathy associated with these infections to persist for 2 months. Serum angiotensin-converting enzyme level is a nonspecific test for sarcoidosis but is also elevated in other granulomatous diseases and is not sensitive or specific enough to be used as an initial diagnostic test. Lymphadenopathy associated with sarcoidosis requires a biopsy for diagnosis. In this patient, an excisional biopsy is necessary primarily to rule out the malignancy, particularly lymphoma.

318. The answer is a. (*Kasper, pp 654–655.*) The staging of Hodgkin's disease is important so that proper treatment can be planned. Stage I (single lymph node bearing area) or stage II (more than one lymph node site on the same side of the diaphragm) patients who have good prognostic features may be treated with radiation therapy. Those with stage III (affected lymph nodes on both sides of the diaphragm) or stage IV (extranodal disease) are treated with combination chemotherapy. A CT scan or an MRI of the abdomen and pelvis will show evidence of lymph node involvement below the diaphragm. Staging laparotomy with splenectomy, formerly done to provide pathology of the periaortic nodes and spleen, is rarely done today. Gallium scans can be useful in difficult cases. Bone marrow biopsy is usually performed to exclude bone marrow disease, which would imply stage IV.

319. The answer is b. (*Kasper, pp 543–550.*) A prostate biopsy is necessary to confirm the diagnosis of prostatic carcinoma. A metastatic workup, including bone scan, would then follow. Bone scan is a very sensitive test for metastatic prostate carcinoma, which tends to spread through the venous plexus surrounding the prostate to the sacrum and lower lumbar vertebrae. Since prostate cancer stimulates osteoblastic activity of the bone, and since osteoblasts (rather than osteoclasts) take up the tracer used in bone scanning, the test is very reliable. Pure osteolytic metastases (typically seen in myeloma, occasionally in thyroid or renal carcinoma) will not produce hot spots on bone scans. MRI scanning of pelvic nodes is occasionally used to assess resectability. If this patient has bony metastases, however, systemic rather than local therapy will be necessary.

320. The answer is d. (*Kasper, pp 543–550.*) Patients with metastatic prostatic carcinoma are treated with endocrine therapy to shrink primary and secondary lesions by depriving prostatic tissue of circulating androgens. Estrogens are no longer recommended because of the high incidence of cardiovascular events. Most patients now receive a GnRH analogue or surgical castration; whether an antiandrogen (such as flutamide) provides additional benefit is currently a matter of debate. Radiotherapy is used for localized disease, but is less effective than hormonal therapy. The survival benefit of chemotherapy, if any, is small.

321. The answer is c. (*Kasper, pp 674–675.*) Heparin is the commonest cause of drug-induced thrombocytopenia. Between 10 and 15% of patients receiving unfractionated heparin develop thrombocytopenia. The drop in platelet count is due to the production of an antibody against a complex of heparin and platelet factor 4. Low-molecular-weight heparin can also cause thrombocytopenia, although less frequently than unfractionated heparin. Although a bone marrow study to show the presence of megakaryocytes is occasionally indicated in unexplained thrombocytopenia, in this patient with a history strongly suggestive of a drug-induced thrombocytopenia, a bone marrow examination would not be necessary. The diagnosis of idiopathic thrombocytopenic purpura requires the exclusion of drugs likely to cause a decline in the platelet count. Other drugs that may cause thrombocytopenia include chemotherapeutic agents, antibiotics such as sulfonamides and β-lactams, and cardiovascular agents including thiazide diuretics or quinidine.

322. The answer is c. (*Kasper, pp 688–689.*) Heparin-induced thrombocytopenia causes a white clot syndrome rather than bleeding (which is uncommon in HIT). The patient develops platelet aggregation and excess clotting, which can be either venous or arterial. Patients may develop stroke, myocardial infarction, digital gangrene, and so on. Although HIT usually resolves spontaneously after 7 to 10 days, the development of thrombosis due to HIT requires therapy with alternative anticoagulants. Although low-molecular-weight heparin infrequently causes HIT, its use is contraindicated in the white clot syndrome. The administration of lepirudin or agatroban (direct thrombin antagonists) can be lifesaving. Warfarin is used long term, but only after lepirudin or danaproid has been instituted. Although the lupus anticoagulant can cause both venous and arterial thrombosis, this patient likely has a drug-induced thrombocytopenia. The lupus anticoagulant often occurs in the absence of clinical lupus; therefore, an ANA would not be indicated.

323. The answer is c. *(Kasper, pp 21–23, 689–692.)* Rifampin induces the cytochrome P450 that metabolizes warfarin; higher doses of warfarin are required to overcome this effect. When rifampin is stopped, the dose of warfarin necessary to produce a therapeutic prothrombin time will decrease. Barbiturates also accelerate the metabolism of warfarin. Many drugs interfere with the metabolism and clearance of warfarin. Drugs such as nonsteroidal anti-inflammatories can compete with warfarin for albumin-binding sites and will lead to an increased prothrombin time. The list of medications that can either increase or decrease the effect of warfarin is long; all patients given this drug should be advised to contact their physician before taking any new drug. They should also be counseled about over-the-counter drugs (aspirin and NSAIDs) or even health food supplements (such as ginkgo biloba) that can also affect the prothrombin time in these patients.

324. The answer is b. *(Kasper, pp 2298–2303.)* Patients with hemochromatosis and cirrhosis have a very high incidence of hepatocellular carcinoma. The incidence of this complication is 30% and increases with age. Weight loss and abdominal pain suggest hepatoma in this patient. A CT scan or ultrasound would be indicated. The picture of right upper quadrant pain and elevated alkaline phosphatase would not suggest acute hepatitis (which causes an elevation of the transaminases) or worsening of the cirrhosis caused by hemochromatosis. Primary biliary cirrhosis can cause an obstructive biliary disease, but would be much less likely in this patient.

325. The answer is c. *(Kasper, pp 195, 443.)* The lesion described is characteristic of leukoplakia. This is a precancerous lesion that requires biopsy. Histologically, these lesions show hyperkeratosis, acanthosis, and atypia.

There are homogeneous and nonhomogeneous types; the homogeneous are much more likely to undergo malignant transformation. Oropharyngeal *Candida* would be unlikely to occur in this patient and would appear as a more diffuse, lacy lesion of the buccal mucosa and oropharynx. The white plaque of thrush would rub off, leaving a slightly erythematous and inflamed mucosa underneath.

326. The answer is a. (*Kasper, pp 517–518.*) A breast mass, even in a young woman, requires evaluation. Although most such masses are benign, breast cancer is still the commonest cause of cancer death in this age group. Risk factor assessment cannot provide sufficient reassurance. Either excisional biopsy or, in selected hands, fine needle aspiration with follow-up, will be needed to detect cases of breast cancer before metastases outside the breast have occurred.

327. The answer is b. (*Kasper, pp 626–631.*) This patient has polycythemia vera, a clonal proliferative disorder of the bone marrow in which all three cell lines (red blood cells, platelets, and myelocytes) are overproduced. The other classic myeloproliferative disorders are chronic myelogenous leukemia, essential thrombocytosis, and myelofibrosis. The myelodysplastic disorders are diseases where red cell production is disordered; white blood cells and platelets are normal, at least initially. These patients present with anemia, often in association with mild macrocytosis and other features of altered marrow maturation (ringed sideroblasts, hypolobulated polys, etc.). Splenomegaly and cellular overproduction are not features of the myelodysplastic syndromes.

328. The answer is c. (*Kasper, pp 593–597.*) Splenomegaly is not typical of sickle cell anemia. Recurrent splenic infarcts usually occur during childhood and lead to a small, infarcted spleen with functional asplenia. These patients often have Howell-Jolly bodies on peripheral blood smear (indicative of asplenia) and have an increased incidence of infection with encapsulated organisms. The presence of an enlarged spleen in a patient with sickle cells on peripheral blood smear is most often seen in hemoglobin SC disease. The state of hemolysis results in an unconjugated hyperbilirubinemia and low-grade icterus. Anemia and hypoxemia result in a hyperdynamic circulation and a systolic ejection murmur. Ankle ulcers and other chronic skin ulcers may be persistent problems, particularly in those with severe anemia.

3222   Medicine

329. The answer is e. (*Kasper, pp 610–611.*) This patient has developed a hemolytic anemia secondary to an antimalarial drug. Toxins or drugs such as primaquine, sulfamethoxazole, and nitrofurantoin cause hemolysis in patients with G6PD deficiency. It occurs most commonly in African Americans; since the G6PD gene is carried on the X chromosome, most affected patients are males. The drugs that cause hemolysis in G6PD deficiency are oxidizing agents. Oxidant stress on red blood cells is counteracted by reduced glutathione. NADPH (which is required to regenerate reduced glutathione after it has been oxidized) is produced by the hexose monophosphate shunt. G6PD is the first enzyme in this metabolic pathway. If this enzyme is less active, the cell cannot replace GSH and succumbs to oxidizing stress. Clinically this can range from mild to life-threatening hemolysis. In mild cases, no treatment is necessary; once the offending drug is eliminated, the hemolysis resolves.

330. The answer is d. (*Kasper, pp 602–605.*) With anemia and hypersegmented polys, this patient has a megaloblastic anemia. The evidence for neuropathy makes B_{12} deficiency the diagnosis, since folate deficiency does not cause neuropathy. Pernicious anemia with low B_{12} levels and decreased secretion of intrinsic factor is the most likely cause, although B_{12} deficiency from intestinal malabsorption cannot be ruled out. Antiparietal antibody occurs in 90% of patients with pernicious anemia.

331. The answer is b. (*Kasper, pp 631–637.*) The patient has probably had myelodysplastic syndrome (MDS) for years. This is a common cause of anemia with mild macrocytosis in the elderly. Some of these patients will transform into acute myeloid leukemia. The leukemic cells can expand the marrow and cause diffuse bone pain (especially over the sternum and around the knees). Although 20% of patients with MDS can have mild splenomegaly, the newly detected spleen tip and the rapidly worsening pancytopenia suggest that leukemic cells are squeezing out the normal hematopoietic cells. Patients with secondary AML (i.e., AML that arises from a preexisting hematopoietic disease) have a grave prognosis and respond poorly to combination chemotherapy.

332. The answer is b. (*Kasper, pp 683–684.*) This patient with gram-negative bacteremia has developed disseminated intravascular coagulation, as evidenced by multiple-site bleeding, thrombocytopenia, fragmented red blood cells on peripheral smear, prolonged PT and PTT, and reduced fibrinogen levels from depletion of coagulation proteins. Initial treatment is directed at correcting the underlying disorder—in this case infection. Although heparin was formerly recommended for the treatment of DIC, it is now used rarely and only in unusual circumstances (such as acute promyelocytic leukemia). For the patient who continues to bleed, supplementation of platelets and clotting factors (with fresh frozen plasma or cryoprecipitate) may help control life-threatening bleeding. Red cell fragmentation and low platelet count can be seen in microangiopathic disorders such as TTP, but in these disorders the coagulation pathway is not activated. Therefore, in TTP the prothrombin time and partial thromboplastin time as well as the plasma fibrinogen levels will be normal.

333. The answer is c. *(Kasper, p 2115.)* Propylthiouracil can cause a mild leukopenia that does not require discontinuation of the drug. Drug-induced agranulocytosis is a life-threatening complication occurring in 0.1 to 0.2% of patients on antithyroid medications and requires immediate discontinuation of the drug. Agranulocytosis is an immune-mediated disorder; the absolute neutrophil count is often extremely depressed (usually less than 100). Generally the neutrophil count will recover 5 to 7 days after the offending drug has been discontinued. During this time the patient is at grave risk of septicemia. Although blood cultures are indicated in this patient prior to the administration of antibiotics, the most important initial step is evaluating the white blood cell count.

334. The answer is c. *(Kasper, pp 662–667.)* Although the risk of the transmission of infectious agents with transfusions is very low (probably less than one in a million for hepatitis C and HIV), other types of transfusion reactions still occur. Febrile and allergic reactions occur between 1 and 4% of the time. A more serious consequence is transfusion-related acute lung injury (TRALI), a form of noncardiogenic pulmonary edema that, while self-limited, can lead to respiratory failure and the need for mechanical ventilation. It is caused by antibodies in the *donor* plasma that bind to HLA antigens on the patient's white blood cells. Aspiration pneumonia can mimic TRALI but usually has other features (e.g., purulent sputum) to distinguish it.

335. The answer is d. *(Kasper, pp 558–562.)* Although lipomas are the commonest soft tissue mass, they are soft and mobile with the subcutaneous tissue and grow very slowly. Any atypical or enlarging soft tissue mass should be further evaluated, either by CT or MRI scan or by biopsy, because this is how soft tissue sarcomas present. The size, firmness, and fixity to deep tissues are all worrisome features in this patient, and a biopsy should be requested even if the CT scan is reassuring; therefore, open biopsy would be the preferred approach. Sixty percent of soft tissue sarcomas arise in the extremities, with the lower extremities three times as common as the upper extremities. A variety of histological types are possible and are not predictable from clinical features, although malignant fibrous histiocytomas are most common. The only curative approach is complete surgical resection. Radiation and chemotherapy have a role in adjuvant or palliative therapy. Occasional patients with favorable metastatic disease enter long-term remission with aggressive therapy. Soft tissue sarcomas metastasize hematogenously, most often to the lungs; lymph node metastases would not be expected.

336–338. The answers are 336-a, 337-d, 338-b. *(Kasper, pp 498–503, 519–523, 551–553.)* Most cancers are cured only when found in an early or localized state. A few malignancies, however, are curable even when distant metastases are present. Among these are gestational choriocarcinoma, certain acute leukemias, and certain lymphomas. The demonstration that testicular carcinoma is curable by combination chemotherapy represented a major advance in the treatment of this neoplasm. Seminomas are quite sensitive to radiation therapy, but even nonseminomatous tumors are curable with platinum-based chemotherapy. Metastases beyond the retroperitoneal nodes, very high α-fetoprotein or β-HCG levels, or LDH levels above 10 times normal confer poor prognosis, but even these patients can be cured 50% of the time.

Metastatic melanoma is a devastating disease with 5-year survival of less than 10%. The only curative strategy for melanoma is surgery when the disease is localized (preferably to the skin, although 50% of those with one metastatic regional node can be cured with local excision and lymph node dissection). Chemotherapy produces partial response in less than 20% of these patients. Interferon and interleukin 2 are used with similarly disappointing results.

Breast cancer that has metastasized beyond the axillary lymph nodes is an incurable disease; however, many forms of therapy lead to complete remission in 30 to 40% of patients treated. Patients who are estrogen receptor–positive are often treated with hormone-based regimens. ER-negative and younger women usually receive doxorubicin-based treatment. In addition, bone metastases can be palliated with bisphosphonates.

339–341. The answers are 339-a, 340-c, 341-d. *(Kasper, pp 586–592.)* The alcoholic patient being treated for tuberculosis has sideroblastic anemia. Both ethanol and isoniazid inhibit one or more steps in heme synthesis. The disorder results in ringed sideroblasts, nucleated erythroid precursors, a hypochromic microcytic anemia, and a characteristic increase in serum iron and transferrin saturation.

Both iron-deficiency anemia and anemia of chronic disease are associated with a low serum iron level. In iron-deficiency anemia, the TIBC is high and the iron saturation is usually less than 10%. In anemia of chronic disease, the iron-binding capacity is low and the saturation is usually between 10 and 20%. In borderline cases, a serum ferritin level will usually make the distinction (it is low in iron-deficiency anemia and normal or high in anemia of chronic disease). Both anemias can be normocytic if mild and microcytic if moderate in severity. Anemia of chronic disease is rarely severe (i.e., hemoglobin rarely below 8.5); a severe anemia associated with a very low MCV is usually iron deficiency or thalassemia.

The anemia of renal disease is normocytic and normochromic. The red cells themselves are normal but are not stimulated to proliferate due to inadequate amounts of erythropoietin. The diseased kidney is unable to produce adequate amounts of erythropoietin. Numbers of white cells and platelets are usually normal.

342–344. The answers are 342-d, 343-a, 344-b. *(Kasper, pp 566–571.)* The classic Trousseau syndrome consists of migratory superficial thrombophlebitis. A single episode of tenderness and inflammation in a superficial vein is common and usually benign, but recurrent unprovoked episodes should prompt a search for an underlying neoplasm. Cancer of the pancreas is the classic and commonest cancer, but any mucin-producing carcinoma can produce this syndrome.

Humoral hypercalcemia of malignancy resembles hyperparathyroidism, but the substance produced by the cancer is parathormone-related peptide (PTHrP), which does not cross-react with PTH on modern assays. PTHrP is an oncofetal protein involved in squamous differentiation in the fetus. For this reason squamous cancers (lung, head and neck, cervix) are the usual causes. Adenocarcinomas are relatively uncommon causes of this syndrome.

Oat cell (small cell undifferentiated) carcinomas of the lung arise from neuroendocrine cells and thus commonly produce ectopic hormones. ADH (vasopressin) is the commonest and causes hyponatremia, but production of ACTH (usually causing hypokalemia and muscle weakness rather than the classic full-blown Cushing syndrome) occurs frequently. Therefore a lung mass in association with either hyponatremia or hypokalemia suggests oat cell carcinoma.

Neurology

Questions

DIRECTIONS: Each item below contains a question followed by suggested responses. Select the **one best** response to each question.

345. A 30-year-old male complains of unilateral headaches with rhinorrhea and tearing of the eye on the side of the headache. Episodes are precipitated by alcohol. Headaches may become a problem for weeks to months, after which a headache-free period occurs. Which of the following is the most likely diagnosis?

a. Migraine
b. Cluster headache
c. Sinusitis
d. Tension headache

346. A 35-year-old previously healthy woman complains of a severe, excruciating headache and then has a transient loss of consciousness. There are no focal neurologic findings. Which of the following is the best next step in evaluation?

a. CT scan without contrast
b. CT scan with contrast
c. Carotid angiogram
d. Holter monitor

347. A 70-year-old male complains of the sudden onset of syncope. It occurs without warning and with no sweating, dizziness, or light-headedness. He believes episodes tend to occur when he turns his head too quickly or sometimes when he is shaving. The best way to make a definitive diagnosis in this patient is which of the following?

a. ECG
b. Carotid massage with ECG monitoring
c. Holter monitor
d. Electrophysiologic studies to evaluate the AV node

348. A 38-year-old woman is brought to the emergency room by her family. They know that she has recently been in a psychiatric hospital but do not know the diagnosis or her medications. She has been vomiting and taking little by mouth over the past few days. The woman is ataxic and confused. She has a coarse tremor that is more prominent with movement. A moderate-sized diffuse goiter is present. Which of the following treatments is most likely to be beneficial?

a. Gastric lavage and charcoal
b. Intravenous saline
c. Intravenous potassium
d. Parenteral haloperidol

349. A 30-year-old male complains of leg weakness and paresthesias of the arm and leg. Five years previously he had an episode of transient visual loss. On physical exam, there is hyperreflexia, bilateral Babinski signs, and cerebellar dysmetria with poor finger-to-nose movement. When the patient is asked to look to the right, the left eye does not move normally past the midline. Nystagmus is noted in the abducting eye. A more detailed history suggests the patient has had several episodes of gait difficulty that have resolved spontaneously. He appears to be stable between these episodes. He has no systemic symptoms of fever or weight loss. Which of the following is the most appropriate next test to order?

a. Lumbar puncture
b. MRI
c. Quantitative IgG levels
d. Oligoclonal banding

350. A 26-year-old woman presents for follow-up of her multiple sclerosis. She has had two separate episodes of optic neuritis and has noticed stutteringly progressive weakness in her lower extremities. She has a mild neurogenic bladder. MRI scanning reveals several plaques in the periventricular white matter and several other plaques in the brainstem. Which of the following best summarizes the role of interferon β for this disease?

a. It can reduce the number of relapses and the appearance of new lesions on MRI
b. It can cure one-third of patients
c. It improves survival
d. It improves patients' symptoms and has no significant side effects

351. A 76-year-old woman consults you because of leg discomfort. Her legs are comfortable during the day, but in the evening she develops an uncomfortable creepy-crawly sensation that keeps her awake for hours. The feeling is temporarily relieved by movement; she will awaken, pace around, and sometimes run water on her legs to achieve relief. Which of the following is the best initial treatment for her condition?

a. Zolpidem 5 mg po at bedtime
b. Trazodone 50 mg po at bedtime
c. Stretching exercises of the legs
d. Pramipexole 0.125 mg po in the evening

352. A 50-year-old male complains of slowly progressive weakness over several months. Walking has become more difficult, as has using his hands. There are no sensory, bowel, or bladder complaints, or any problems in thinking, speech, or vision. Examination shows distal muscle weakness with muscle wasting and fasciculations. There are also upper motor neuron signs, including extensor plantar reflexes and hyperreflexia in wasted muscle groups. Which of the following laboratory tests is most likely to be abnormal in this patient?

a. Cerebrospinal fluid white blood cell count
b. Sensory conduction studies
c. CT scan of the brain
d. Electromyography

353. A 73-year-old woman develops increasing muscle weakness without sensory symptoms. She is mildly hyperreflexic but also has muscle wasting and fasciculations. The possibility of an atypical cervical radiculopathy is entertained, but an MRI scan of the cervical spine shows no cord or nerve root involvement. A diagnosis of amyotrophic lateral sclerosis is made, and riluzole 100 mg daily is prescribed. After discovering that the medication is very expensive, the patient returns and requests more information about her treatment. Which of the following statements about riluzole is true?

a. Riluzole arrests the underlying pathologic process in ALS
b. Riluzole was FDA-approved for ALS because it improves survival rate
c. Riluzole has no significant side effects
d. Insulin-like growth factor is another alternative for the treatment of ALS

354. A 20-year-old woman complains of weakness that is worse in the afternoon, worse during repetitive activity, and improved by rest. When fatigued, the patient is unable to hold her head up, speak, or chew her food. On physical exam, there is no loss of reflexes, sensation, or coordination. Which of the following is the underlying pathogenesis of this disease?

a. Serum antiacetylcholine receptor antibodies causing neuromuscular transmission failure
b. Destruction of anterior horn cells by virus
c. Progressive muscular atrophy
d. Demyelinating disease

355. A 46-year-old man notices diplopia in the afternoon or when he is particularly tired. Sometimes his muscles feel weak and he has difficulty lifting heavy objects, but the symptoms resolve promptly with rest. The diagnosis of myasthenia gravis is made by a positive edrophonium test, repetitive nerve stimulation test of a weak muscle, and antiacetylcholine receptor antibody assay. MRI of the mediastinum is now indicated to do which of the following?

a. Rule out tuberculosis before starting prednisone
b. Rule out thymoma
c. Look for small cell carcinoma and Lambert-Eaton syndrome
d. Rule out sarcoidosis

356. Three weeks after an upper respiratory illness, a 25-year-old male develops weakness of his arms and legs over several days. On physical exam he is tachypneic, with shallow respirations and symmetric muscle weakness in both arms and legs. There is no obvious sensory deficit, but motor reflexes cannot be elicited. Which of the following is the most likely diagnosis?

a. Myasthenia gravis
b. Multiple sclerosis
c. Guillain-Barré syndrome
d. Dermatomyositis
e. Diabetes mellitus

357. A 56-year-old woman develops difficulty ambulating several weeks after receiving an influenza vaccine. She is found to have distal muscle weakness and areflexia in the lower extremities. During a 2-day observation period the weakness ascends, and she begins to notice weakness of the hands. She notices mild tingling, but the sensory examination is normal. The diagnosis of Guillain-Barré syndrome is strongly suspected. The workup of this patient is most likely to show which of the following?

a. Acellular spinal fluid with high protein
b. Abnormal EMG that shows axonal degeneration
c. Positive Tensilon test
d. Elevated CPK
e. Respiratory alkalosis by arterial blood gases

358. A 76-year-old woman presents with numbness and mild weakness in the legs. She has noticed mild numbness in the fingertips bilaterally. The symptoms have been slowly progressive over the past year. She rarely goes to the doctor and takes no medications. Neurological exam shows sensory loss to light touch to the knees and wrists in a symmetric pattern. Joint position sensation is less severely affected. Ankle reflexes are absent and she has mild distal weakness. Which of the following is the most likely abnormality on laboratory testing?

a. Hyperglycemia
b. Macrocytic anemia with a low vitamin B_{12} level
c. Positive ELISA test for HIV
d. Low T_4, elevated TSH

359. A 68-year-old man with a history of hypertension and coronary artery disease presents with right-sided weakness, sensory loss, and an expressive aphasia. Neuroimaging studies are shown. In the emergency department the patient's blood pressure is persistently 160/95. Which of the following is the best next step in management?

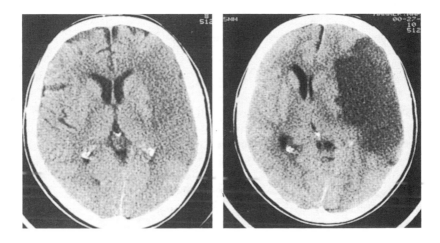

   a. Administer IV nitropruside
   b. Administer oral clonidine 0.1 mg po until the blood pressure drops below 140/90.
   c. Observe the blood pressure
   d. Administer IV mannitol

360. A 45-year-old woman presents to her physician with an 8-month history of gradually increasing limb weakness. She first noticed difficulty climbing stairs, then problems rising from chairs, walking more than half a block, and, finally, lifting her arms above shoulder level. Aside from some difficulty swallowing, she has no ocular, bulbar, or sphincter problems and no sensory complaints. Family history is negative for neurological disease. Examination reveals significant proximal limb and neck muscle weakness with minimal atrophy, normal sensory findings, and intact deep tendon reflexes. Which of the following is the most likely diagnosis in this patient?

a. Polymyositis
b. Cervical myelopathy
c. Myasthenia gravis
d. Mononeuropathy multiplex
e. Limb-girdle muscular dystrophy

361. A 55-year-old diabetic woman suddenly develops weakness of the left side of her face as well as of her right arm and leg. She also has diplopia on left lateral gaze. The responsible lesion is probably located in which of the following?

a. Right cerebral hemisphere
b. Left cerebral hemisphere
c. Right side of the brainstem
d. Left side of the brainstem
e. Right median longitudinal fasciculus

362. A 40-year-old woman complains of headache associated with visual disturbance. Which of the following histories suggests migraine headache as a likely diagnosis?

a. Numbness or tingling of the left face, lips, and hand lasting for 5 to 15 min, followed by throbbing headache
b. An increasingly throbbing headache associated with unilateral visual loss and generalized muscle aches
c. A continuous headache associated with sleepiness, nausea, ataxia, and incoordination of the right upper limb
d. An intense left retroorbital headache associated with transient left-sided ptosis and rhinorrhea
e. A visual field defect that persists following cessation of a unilateral headache

363. A 60-year-old man with Parkinson's disease is receiving levodopa/carbidopa therapy and complains of uncontrollable facial movements. Which of the following is correct?

a. Limb and facial dyskinesias are unusual side effects of chronic levodopa therapy
b. Levodopa treatment, while ameliorating symptoms, does not alter the natural history of the disease
c. Bromocriptine works by increasing the release of dopamine from the substantia nigra
d. Trihexyphenidyl and benztropine mesylate have minimal side effects in the elderly

364. A 72-year-old woman is found unconscious at home by her daughter. In the emergency room the patient does not respond to verbal or noxious stimuli. Which of the following is the most likely cause of her condition?

a. Hypoglycemia
b. Left posterior cerebral artery occlusion
c. Lacunar infarct in the right internal capsule
d. Middle cerebral artery occlusion

365. A 37-year-old factory worker develops increasing weakness in the legs; coworkers have noted episodes of transient confusion. The patient has bilateral foot drop and atrophy; mild wrist weakness is also present. His CBC shows an anemia with a hemoglobin of 9.6 g/dL; examination of the peripheral blood smear shows basophilic stippling. Which of the following is the most likely cause of this patient's symptoms?

a. Amyotrophic lateral sclerosis
b. Lead poisoning
c. Overuse syndrome
d. Myasthenia gravis

DIRECTIONS: Each group of questions below consists of lettered options followed by a set of numbered items. For each numbered item, select the **one** lettered option with which it is **most** closely associated. Each lettered option may be used once, more than once, or not at all.

Questions 366–368

Match the clinical description with the most likely disease process.
a. Parkinson's disease
b. Wilson's disease
c. Huntington's disease
d. Dystonia
e. Essential tremor
f. Tic

366. An 18-year-old male who is admitted to the hospital because of psychotic behavior is found to have a proximal "wing-beating" tremor, dystonia, and incoordination. Serun transaminases are moderately elevated; brownish corneal deposits are noted on slit-lamp exam.

367. An elderly woman notes a tremor associated with slowness of movements and a feeling of gait instability over the past 6 months. The tremor is a slow (3 per second) resting tremor that does not interfere with fine movements.

368. A 37-year-old man is brought to the doctor by his family because of a rapid intellectual decline over the past 2 months. Exam reveals slow writhing movements with dystonic posturing. His father died of a similar illness.

Questions 369–371

For each of the clinical descriptions, select the most likely diagnosis.

a. Senile dementia of the Alzheimer's type
b. Multi-infarct dementia
c. Vitamin B_{12} deficiency
d. Dementia with Lewy bodies
e. Creutzfeldt-Jakob disease
f. Normal pressure hydrocephalus

369. An 80-year-old develops steady, progressive memory and cognitive deficit over 2 years. He has normal blood pressure and no focal neurologic findings, and workup for "treatable" causes of dementia is negative.

370. A 70-year-old male with history of hypertension and diabetes presents with a stepwise loss of intellectual function. Prior episodes have been associated with unilateral weakness and difficulty swallowing. A unilateral Babinski sign is found on neurological exam

371. A 50-year-old presents with rapidly progressive change in mental status over 3 months. Numerous myoclonic jerks accompany the dementia; the EEG shows repetitive high-voltage polyphasic discharges

Questions 372–373

Match each clinical description with the correct diagnosis.

a. Pneumococcal meningitis
b. Cryptococcal meningitis
c. Coxsackievirus (aseptic) meningitis
d. Pyogenic brain abscess
e. Listeria monocytogenes meningitis
f. Herpes simplex encephalitis
g. Cerebral cysticercosis

372. A 50-year-old woman is on high-dose corticosteroids and immuno-suppressives because of renal transplant rejection. She presents with a 10-day history of fever, headache, and confusion. Lumbar puncture reveals 25 lymphocytes/μL and a very high CSF protein. India ink stain is positive.

373. A 28-year-old alcoholic has recently been treated for lung abscess. Three days before this admission, the patient develops headache, fever, and mild right-sided weakness. His MRI scan is shown below.

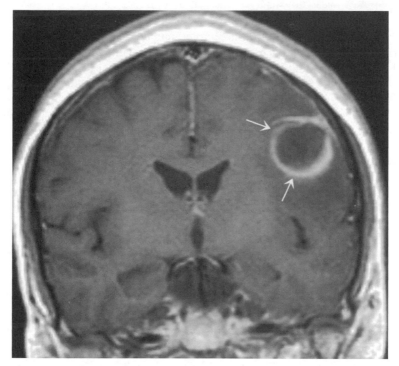

(*Reproduced, with permission, from Kasper DL et al. Harrison's* Principles of Internal Medicine, *16th ed. New York: McGraw-Hill, 2005.*)

Questions 374–376

Match each symptom or sign with the appropriate diagnosis.
a. Tension headache
b. Cluster headache
c. Migraine headache
d. Temporal arteritis
e. Brain tumor
f. Sinusitis
g. Temporomandibular joint dysfunction
h. Tic doloureux

374. A 42-year-old executive complains of a bandlike tightness across the temples and neck, worse in the afternoon, usually relieved by aspirin or acetaminophen. Neurological exam is normal.

375. A 33-year-old man complains of episodes of severe unilateral headache. The pain is localized to one cheekbone and is described as "like an icepick." Each headache lasts 30 to 60 min but may recur several times a day; walking around helps the pain somewhat. He notices lacrimation of the eye on the affected side, usually associated with clear rhinorrhea.

376. An 82-year-old woman complains of worsening headaches and episodes of transient visual loss and diplopia. When she chews, her jaw muscles ache until she stops chewing. Exam reveals a tender nodular right temporal artery. She has a mild normocytic anemia; sedimentation rate is 95.

Questions 377–378

For each symptom, select the most likely type of seizure.
a. Absence (petit mal) seizure
b. Complex partial seizure
c. Simple partial seizure
d. Atonic seizure
e. Myoclonic seizure

377. The patient recalls having episodes where he smells a pungent odor, becomes sweaty, and loses consciousness. His wife describes a period of motor arrest followed by repetitive picking movements that last about a minute. The patient does not fall or lose muscle control.

378. The teacher of a 14-year-old child recounts episodes where the child stares into space and does not respond to verbal commands for a few seconds. These episodes occur several times per day. An EEG shows 3-per-second spike and slow wave discharges.

Questions 379–382

For each symptom of cerebrovascular disease, select the site of the lesion.

a. Internal carotid artery
b. Middle cerebral artery
c. Midbasilar artery
d. Anterior cerebral artery
e. Penetrating branch, middle cerebral artery

379. An elderly man has noticed three episodes of visual loss in his right eye. The vision in that eye goes black "like somebody pulling down a window shade." The symptom lasts 20 to 30 min and resolves promptly. Between episodes he feels well.

380. A 75-year-old hypertensive woman presents with whirling vertigo, nausea, and weakness on the right side of her body. On exam she has nystagmus, left facial sensory loss, and right arm and leg weakness.

381. A 37-year-old smoker who takes birth control pills presents with sudden weakness and numbness of the right side of her body. She has a severe expressive aphasia and tends to neglect the deficit on her right side.

382. A 79-year-old diabetic presents with right-sided weakness. The weakness is equal in the right face, arm, and leg. Sensation, speech, and comprehension are intact.

Neurology

Answers

345. The answer is b. *(Kasper, pp 85–94.)* This headache is most consistent with a type of neurovascular headache called cluster headache. These occur most often in young men; have a characteristic periodicity, or cluster; and cause lacrimation, nasal stuffiness, and sometimes conjunctival inflammation. Migraines tend not to come and go in this manner, are more throbbing, and are more likely to be associated with nausea and vomiting. Sinusitis is usually bilateral with associated fever and purulent discharge. Tension headaches are usually described as bandlike, without lacrimation or nasal congestion.

346. The answer is a. *(Kasper, pp 2387–2390.)* An excruciating headache with syncope requires evaluation for subarachnoid hemorrhage. In about 80% of patients, there will be enough blood to be visualized on a noncontrast CT scan. If the scan is normal, a lumbar puncture is the next step to establish the presence of subarachnoid blood. A contrast CT scan sometimes obscures the diagnosis because, in an enhanced scan, normal arteries may be mistaken for clotted blood.

347. The answer is b. *(Kasper, pp 126–130.)* When syncope occurs in an older patient as a result of head turning, wearing a tight shirt collar, or shaving over the neck area, carotid sinus hypersensitivity should be considered. It usually occurs in men above the age of 50. Baroreceptors of the carotid sinus are activated and pass impulses through the glossopharyngeal nerve to the medulla oblongata. Some consider the process to be quite rare. Gentle massage of one carotid sinus at a time may show a period of asystole. This should be performed in a controlled setting with monitoring and atropine available.

348. The answer is b. *(Kasper, pp 2414, 2557.)* This patient is likely to have lithium intoxication. Although many drug intoxications can cause confusion and ataxia, lithium causes a prominent tremor. In addition, because of its effect on iodide uptake, lithium often causes a goiter and occasionally causes hypothyroidism. Lithium is transported in the body like sodium; when the patient becomes volume-depleted, lithium is avidly reabsorbed in the renal tubule and the blood level rises. Treatment is based on the serum lithium level. Mild intoxications are treated with discontinuation of the drug and saline infusion. Life-threatening toxicity requires hemodialysis.

349. The answer is b. *(Kasper, pp 2461–2471.)* This patient's episode of transient blindness was likely due to optic neuritis. This transient loss of vision in one eye occurs in about 25 to 40% of multiple sclerosis patients. (A similar presentation can occur in SLE, sarcoidosis, or syphilis.) In addition, the patient gives a history of a relapsing-remitting process. There are abnormal signs of cerebellar and upper motor neuron disease. Signs and symptoms therefore suggest multiple lesions, making multiple sclerosis the most likely diagnosis. All patients with suspected multiple sclerosis should have an MRI of the brain. MRI is sensitive in defining demyelinating lesions in the brain and spinal cord. Disease-related changes are found in more than 95% of patients who have definite evidence for MS. Most patients do not need lumbar puncture or spinal fluid analysis for diagnosis, although 70% have elevated IgG levels, and myelin basic protein does appear in the CSF during exacerbations. When the diagnosis is in doubt, lumbar puncture is indicated. Pleocytosis of greater than 75 cells per microliter or finding polymorphonuclear leukocytes in the CSF makes the diagnosis of MS unlikely. In some cases, chronic infection such as with syphilis or HIV may be in the differential of MS. Quantitative IgG levels would not be specific enough for diagnosis. Oligoclonal banding of CSF IgG is determined by agarose gel electrophoresis. Two or more bands are found in 70 to 90% of patients with MS.

350. The answer is a. *(Kasper, pp 2461–2471.)* Both interferon β-1b and interferon β-1a are approved for use in patients with multiple sclerosis who have relapsing-remitting or progressive MS. Glatiramer acetate (Copaxone) is now also approved for MS. While patients who receive any one of these treatments have 30% fewer exacerbations and fewer new MRI lesions, the treatments do not cure the disease, and the long-term efficacy is unknown. Interferon β can cause side effects, particularly a flulike syndrome that resolves within several months. MS is rarely the direct cause of mortality in patients. Death usually occurs as a result of a complication of MS, such as infection in a debilitated patient.

351. The answer is d. *(Kasper, p 158.)* This woman has restless legs syndrome, a common sensory complaint in the elderly. It is characterized by ill-defined leg discomfort that occurs in the evening when the patient is reclining or at night when the patient is trying to sleep. The uncomfortable sensation is relieved by movement. Exam is normal or shows at most a mild distal sensory loss. There are no motor or reflex changes. Although most often idiopathic, RLS can be asociated with iron deficiency or renal insufficiency. Although several agents (benzodiazepines, opioids) can provide symptomatic relief, dopamine-enhancing drugs are most effective. Levodopa-carbidopa is effective, but may lead to rebound effects, so direct dopamine agonists (pramipexole, pergolide, ropinirole) are now preferred.

352. The answer is d. *(Kasper, pp 2424–2428.)* The disease described involves motor neurons exclusively. Amyotrophic lateral sclerosis affects both upper and lower motor neurons. In this patient, there is upper and lower motor neuron involvement without sensory deficit. Lower motor neuron signs include focal weakness, focal wasting, and fasciculations. Upper motor neuron signs include an extensor plantar response and an increased tendon reflex in a weakened muscle. Peripheral neuropathy and dementia do not occur in ALS. Primary muscle diseases produce weakness by affecting muscle fibers without interfering with the nerve itself or the neuromuscular junction. Muscular dystrophy, polymyositis, and the neuromuscular junction disorder myesthenia gravis cause (usually proximal) muscle weakness but not the atrophy and upper motor neuron signs seen in this patient. EMG would show widespread denervation and fibrillation potentials with preserved nerve conduction velocities. Sensory neurons are normal. There is no inflammatory reaction in the CSF. A CT or an MRI of the brain may be necessary to rule out a mass in the region of the foramen magnum. In some patients, a CT of the cervical spine might be needed to rule out a structural lesion of the spine, which could mimic ALS.

353. The answer is b. *(Kasper, pp 2214–2428.)* Riluzole is approved by the FDA for the treatment of ALS. It has been shown to moderately prolong life in the ALS patient, although it does not arrest the disease process. Its mechanism of action may be inhibition of the release of the neurotransmitter glutamate with reduction of excitotoxicity. The drug has several side effects, including nausea, weight loss, and liver function abnormalities. Insulin-like growth factor (IGF-1) was shown to slow the progression of

ALS in one study, but results were not confirmed in a second study, and IGF-1 is not available as a treatment option at present.

354. The answer is a. *(Kasper, pp 2518–2523.)* The disease process described is myasthenia gravis, a neuromuscular disease marked by muscle weakness and fatigability. Myasthenia gravis results from a reduction in the number of junctional acetylcholine receptors as a result of autoantibodies. Antibodies cross-link these receptors, causing a facilitation of endocytosis and degradation in lysosomes. A decreased number of available acetylcholine receptors results in decreased efficiency of neuromuscular transmission. Successive nerve impulses result in the activation of fewer muscle fibers and produce fatigue. Myasthenia presents with weakness and fatigability, particularly of cranial muscles, causing diplopia, ptosis, nasal speech, and dysarthria. Asymmetric limb weakness also occurs.

355. The answer is b. *(Kasper, p 2522.)* Ten percent of myasthenia patients have thymic tumors. Surgical removal of all thymomas is necessary because of local tumor spread. Even in the absence of tumor, 85% of patients clinically improve after thymectomy. It is now consensus that thymectomy be performed in all patients with generalized MG who are between puberty and age 55. Sarcoidosis causes peripheral neuropathy and aseptic meningitis, but not a myasthenia syndrome. Small cell carcinoma is associated with Lambert-Eaton syndrome, a paraneoplastic syndrome similar to myasthenia. In Lambert-Eaton syndrome, an autoimmune response results in anti–calcium channel antibodies. A chest x-ray would be sufficient to screen for malignancy or infection.

356. The answer is c. *(Kasper, pp 2513–2518.)* This patient presents with an acute symmetrical polyneuropathy characteristic of Guillain-Barré syndrome. This demyelinating disease is often preceded by a viral illness. Characteristically, there is little sensory involvement, and about 30% of patients require ventilatory assistance. Loss of deep tendon reflexes, especially in the lower extremities, is an important clue to the lower motor neuron involvement that characterizes GBS. Dermatomyositis usually presents insidiously with proximal muscle weakness. Myasthenia gravis also presents insidiously with muscle weakness worsened by repetitive use. Diplopia, ptosis, and facial weakness are common first complaints. Reflexes would be preserved in those diseases that affect muscle and not peripheral nerves. Multiple sclerosis causes demyelinating lesions disseminated in time and space and would not occur in this acute, symmetrical manner. Diabetes mellitus can cause a variety of neuropathies, but would not be rapidly progressive as in this patient.

357. The answer is a. *(Kasper, pp 2513–2518.)* Guillain-Barré syndrome is characterized by an elevated CSF protein with few if any white blood cells. EMG would show a demyelinating process with nonuniform slowing and conduction block. Arterial blood gases would show a respiratory acidosis secondary to hypoventilation. CPK levels should be normal, as there is no involvement of muscle in this disease process. Research laboratories show antiganglioside antibodies in as high as 50% of patients with Guillain-Barré syndrome.

358. The answer is a. *(Kasper, pp 2503–2510.)* The insidious onset of a distal and progressive sensory loss is characteristic of diabetic neuropathy. In many metabolic neuropathies, the longest nerve fibers are affected first, leading to the stocking-glove pattern of sensory loss. Autonomic changes can accompany the sensory loss. Some diabetics will have vascular changes in the vasa nervorum which can lead to asymmetric peripheral or cranial neuropathies; these are often reversible while the distal neuropathy is usually progressive. It is not rare for neuropathy to be a presenting symptom of type 2 diabetes, particularly if the patient has not had prior glucose testing. Other conditions often associated with peripheral neuropathy include medication side effects, toxins, uremia, neoplasms, vitamin deficiency, and amyloidosis. EMG and nerve conduction velocity testing separate neuropathy into axonal and demyelinating varieties and often provide important diagnostic information.

359. The answer is c. *(Kasper, pp 2374–2387.)* Although hypertension is an important cause of stroke, it should not be aggressively treated in the setting of acute cerebral ischemia. Since cerebral autoregulation is disrupted in acute stroke, a drop in blood pressure can decrease perfusion and worsen the so-called ischemic penumbra. Generally, blood pressure of less than 185/110 is not treated. Many specialists recommend more aggressive blood pressure control in acute hemorrhagic stroke, however.

360. The answer is a. *(Kasper, pp 2540–2545.)* Polymyositis is an acquired myopathy characterized by subacute symmetrical weakness of proximal limb and trunk muscles that progresses over several weeks or months. When a characteristic skin rash occurs, the disease is known as dermatomyositis. In addition to progressive proximal limb weakness, the patient often presents with dysphagia and neck muscle weakness. Up to half of cases with polymyositis-dermatomyositis may have, in addition, features of connective tissue diseases (rheumatoid arthritis, lupus erythematosus, scleroderma, Sjögren syndrome). Laboratory findings include an elevated serum CK level, an EMG showing myopathic potentials with fibrillations, and a muscle biopsy showing necrotic muscle fibers and inflammatory infiltrates. Polymyositis is clinically distinguished from the muscular dystrophies by its less prolonged course and lack of family history. It is distinguished from myasthenia gravis by its lack of ocular muscle involvement, absence of variability in strength over hours or days, and lack of response to cholinesterase inhibitor drugs.

361. The answer is d. (*Kasper, pp 2381–2387.*) This patient has weakness of the left face and the contralateral (right) arm and leg, commonly called a *crossed hemiplegia*. Such crossed syndromes are characteristic of brainstem lesions. In this case, the lesion is an infarct localized to the left inferior pons caused by occlusion of a branch of the basilar artery. The infarct has damaged the left sixth and seventh cranial nerves or nuclei in the left pons with resultant diplopia on left lateral gaze and left facial weakness. Also damaged in the left pons is the left corticospinal tract, proximal to its decussation in the medulla; this damage causes weakness in the right arm and leg. This classic presentation is called the Millard-Gubler syndrome.

362. The answer is a. (*Kasper, pp 85–94.*) The differential diagnosis of headaches associated with neurological or visual dysfunction is important because it encompasses a variety of disorders, some quite serious and others relatively benign. Classic (or neurological) migraine is generally a familial disorder that begins in childhood or early adult life. Typically, the onset of an episode is marked by the progression of a neurological disturbance over 5 to 15 min, followed by a unilateral (or occasionally bilateral) throbbing headache for several hours up to a day. The most common neurological disturbance involves formed or unformed flashes of light that impair vision in one of the visual fields (scintillating scotoma). Other possible neurological symptoms include numbness and tingling of the unilateral face, lips, and hand; weakness of an arm or leg; mild aphasia; and mental confusion. The transience of the neurological symptoms distinguishes migraine from other, more serious conditions that cause headaches. Persistence of a visual field defect, speech disturbance, or mild hemiparesis suggests a focal lesion (e.g., arteriovenous malformation with hemorrhage or infarct). In the case of persistent ataxia, limb incoordination, and nausea, one should consider a posterior fossa (possibly cerebellar) mass lesion. Monocular visual loss in an elderly patient with throbbing headaches should initiate a search for cranial (temporal) arteritis. This should include a sedimentation rate (usually elevated) and a temporal artery biopsy (which would show a giant cell arteritis). Fifty percent of these patients have the generalized muscle aches seen with polymyalgia rheumatica. Unilateral orbital or retroorbital headaches that occur nightly for a period of 2 to 8 weeks are characteristic of cluster headaches. These headaches are often associated with ipsilateral injection of the conjunctivum, nasal stuffiness, rhinorrhea, and, less commonly, miosis, ptosis, and cheek edema. Although both migraine and cluster headaches may respond to treatment with ergotamine, they are generally considered to be distinct entities.

363. The answer is b. (*Kasper, pp 2406–2413.*) Parkinson's disease (PD) is marked by depletion of dopamine-rich cells in the substantia nigra. The resulting decrease in striatal dopamine is the basis for the classic symptoms of rigidity, bradykinesia, and tremor. By far the most widely used treatment for PD has been levodopa. Levodopa is converted to dopamine in the substantia nigra and then transported to the striatum, where it stimulates dopamine receptors. This is the basis for the drug's clinical effect on PD. Levodopa is usually administered with carbidopa (a decarboxylase inhibitor) in one pill (Sinemet), which prevents levodopa's destruction in the blood and allows it to be given at a dose that is lower and less likely to cause nausea and vomiting. The major problems with levodopa have been (1) significant limb and facial dyskinesias in most patients on chronic therapy and (2) the fact that levodopa treats PD only symptomatically, and the disease process of neuronal loss in the substantia nigra continues despite drug treatment. Other drugs can be used in the treatment of PD. Anticholinergic agents, such as trihexyphenidyl (Artane) and benztropine mesylate (Cogentin), work by restoring the balance between striatal dopamine and acetylcholine. They can have significant anticholinergic effects on the CNS, including confusional states and hallucinations. Bromocriptine and pergolide are dopamine agonists that work directly by stimulating dopamine receptors in the striatum; side effects of these drugs are similar to those of levodopa. Selegiline (Eldepryl) is a selective monoamine oxidase-B (MAO-B) inhibitor that blocks the breakdown of intracerebral dopamine.

364. The answer is a. (*Kasper, pp 1624–1631.*) Focal disorders of the cerebral hemisphere do not cause coma unless the brainstem is compressed by edema or mass effect. Coma implies either severe metabolic derangement of the brain (i.e., hypoglycemia, hyponatremia, intoxication), brainstem dysfunction (affecting the reticular-activating system of the pons), or else bilateral hemispheric insults. Posterior cerebral artery occlusion will cause an occipital lobe infarction with homonymous hemianopsia but should not affect the level of consciousness. Similarly, a lacunar infarct will cause a pure motor or pure sensory stroke but not global brain dysfunction. Although the patient with a middle cerebral artery stroke may be unable to speak, she should be awake and alert.

365. The answer is b. (*Kasper, pp 2577–2579.*) Lead poisoning often causes a peripheral neuropathy with primary motor involvement. It can superficially resemble ALS, but upper motor neuron signs are not seen in lead poisoning. In addition the cognitive changes of lead encephalopathy are not seen in ALS, in peripheral nerve injuries (e.g., carpal or tarsal tunnel syndromes), or in myasthenia. The presence of any anemia in a patient with perpheral neuropathy should prompt the search for an underlying cause. Lead lines may be seen at the gingiva-tooth border. Laboratory testing focuses on protoporphyrin levels (free erythrocyte or zinc) and blood lead levels. Industries often associated with lead exposure include battery and ceramic manufacturing, the demolition of lead-painted houses and bridges, plumbing, soldering, and, occasionally, exposure to the combustion of leaded fuels.

366–368. The answers are 366-b, 367-a, 368-c. (*Kasper, pp 2406–2418.*) A movement disorder in itself in a young person suggests Wilson's disease. This is an autosomal recessive disorder in cellular copper transport that results in copper deposition in tissue. Copper deposition in the basal ganglia causes tremor and rigidity. Copper deposition in the eye

talking or responding, often displays eye fluttering, and commonly shows automatisms such as lip smacking and fumbling movements of the fingers. Attacks end in 2 to 10 seconds with the patient fully alert and able to resume activities. The characteristic EEG abnormality associated with attacks is 3-per-second spike-and-wave activity.

379–382. The answers are 379-a, 380-c, 381-b, 382-e. *(Kasper, pp 167–170, 2381–2387.)* Sudden, painless monocular blindness is a sign of carotid disease. The symptom is also called *amaurosis fugax.* The patient may describe a shade dropping in front of the eye or may describe vision as similar to looking through ground glass. If a thrombus propagates up the carotid to the middle cerebral artery, then symptoms seen in middle cerebral artery occlusion or embolization (hemiparesis with sensory symptoms, aphasia depending on hemispheric dominance) will also occur.

Midbasilar artery disease produces weakness and sensory loss with diplopia, loss of facial sensation or movement, and ataxia. Branches of the basilar artery supply the base of the pons and superior cerebellum. The symptoms described suggest disease in the posterior circulation, which includes paired vertebral arteries, the basilar artery, and the paired posterior cerebral arteries. The basilar artery supplies the cerebellum, medulla, pons, midbrain, thalamus, and temporal and occipital lobes. A midbasilar artery occlusion could cause ataxia of limbs by involving pontine nuclei; paralysis of the face, arm, and leg by involving corticospinal tracts; and impairment of facial sensation by involvement of fifth nerve nucleus.

Occlusion of the entire middle cerebral artery results in contralateral hemiplegia, hemianesthesia, and homonymous hemianopsia. When the dominant hemisphere is involved, aphasia is present. When the nondominant hemisphere is involved, apraxia and neglect are produced. When only a penetrating branch of the middle cerebral artery is affected, the syndrome of pure motor hemiplegia is produced, as the infarct involves only the posterior limb of the internal capsule, involving only motor fibers to the face, arm, and leg (lacunar infarct).

Dermatology

Questions

DIRECTIONS: Each item below contains a question followed by suggested responses. Select the **one best** response to each question.

383. A 20-year-old woman complains of skin problems and is noted to have erythematous papules on her face with blackheads (open comedones) and whiteheads (closed comedones). She has also had cystic lesions. She is prescribed a topical tretinoin (Retin-A), but without a totally acceptable result. Which of the following is correct?

a. Intralesional triamcinolone should be avoided due to its systemic effects
b. Systemically administered isotretinoin therapy cannot be considered unless concomitant contraceptive therapy is provided
c. Antimicrobial therapy is of no value since bacteria are not part of the pathogenesis of the process
d. Isotretinoin is without important side effects as long as it is not used in sexually active women

384. A 22-year-old male presents with a 6-month history of a red, non-pruritic rash over the trunk, scalp, elbows, and knees. These eruptions are more likely to occur during stressful periods and have occurred at sites of skin injury. On exam, sharply demarcated plaques are seen with a thick scale (see photo below). Which of the following statements is correct?

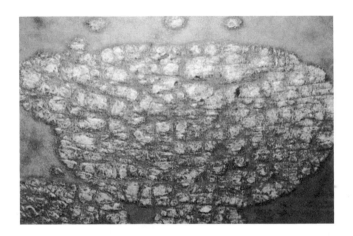

a. The lesions are contagious and contact should be carefully avoided
b. The patient is allergic to metals
c. The clinical description is most consistent with psoriasis
d. The rash is unrelated to stress

385. A 25-year-old complains of fever and myalgias for 5 days and now has developed a macular rash over his palms and soles with some petechial lesions. The patient recently returned from a summer camping trip in the Great Smoky Mountains. Which of the following is the most likely cause of the rash?

a. Contact dermatitis
b. Sexual exposure
c. Tick exposure
d. Contaminated stream

386. A 17-year-old female presents with a pruritic rash localized to the wrist. Papules and vesicles are noted in a bandlike pattern, with slight oozing from some lesions. Which of the following is the most likely cause of the rash?

a. Herpes simplex
b. Shingles
c. Contact dermatitis
d. Seborrheic dermatitis

387. A 35-year-old woman develops an itchy rash over her back, legs, and trunk several hours after swimming in a lake. Erythematous, edematous papules are noted. The wheals vary in size. There are no mucosal lesions and no swelling of the lips (see photo below). Which of the following is the most likely diagnosis?

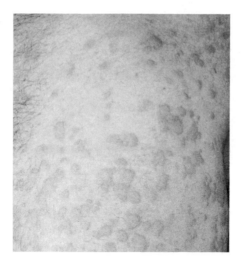

a. Urticaria
b. Folliculitis
c. Erythema multiforme
d. Erythema chronicum migrans

388. A 20-year-old male who enjoys gardening has had repeated episodes of urticaria, which appear to be related to working in his garden. He presents again with itchy, erythematous papules. There is no angioedema or anaphylaxis. Which of the following is the best management approach?

a. Epinephrine
b. Intravenous glucocorticoids
c. Antihistamines and avoidance of offending agent
d. Aspirin

389. A 30-year-old black female has had a history of cough, and a chest x-ray shows bilateral hilar lymphadenopathy. A biopsy shows noncaseating granuloma. Which of the following skin lesions is most consistent with the patient's diagnosis?

a. Seborrheic keratosis
b. Asymmetric pigmented lesion with irregular border
c. Erythema nodosum
d. Umbilicated, dome-shaped yellow papules

390. An elderly homeless male is evaluated for anemia. On exam, he has purpura and ecchymoses of the legs. Perifollicular papules and perifollicular hemorrhages are also noted. There is swelling and bleeding of gums around the patient's teeth as well as tenderness around a hematoma of the calf. Which of the following is the most likely diagnosis?

a. Elder abuse
b. Scurvy
c. Pellagra
d. Beriberi

391. A 53-year-old female presents to the clinic with an erythematous lesion on the dorsum of her right hand. She explains that the lesion has been present for the past 7 months and has not responded to corticosteroid treatment. She is also concerned because the lesion occasionally bleeds and has grown in size during the past few months. On physical exam you notice an 11-mm erythematous plaque with a small central ulceration. The skin is also indurated with mild crusting on the surface. Which of the following is true about this finding?

a. It is a malignant neoplasm of the keratinocytes with the potential to metastasize
b. It is an allergic reaction resulting from the elevation of serum IgE
c. It is a chronic inflammatory condition, which can be complicated by arthritis of small and medium-sized joints
d. It is a malignant neoplasm of the melanocytes with the potential to metastasize
e. It is the most common skin cancer

392. A 50-year-old woman develops pink macules and papules on her hands and forearms in association with a sore throat. The lesions are target-like, with the centers a dusky violet (see photo). A diagnosis of erythema multiforme is made. The most important information obtained from this patient's history is which of the following?

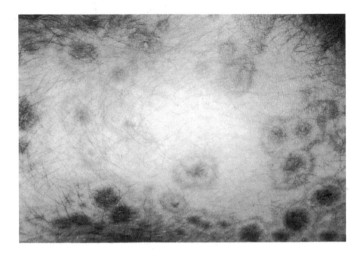

a. The patient has been using tampons
b. The patient is taking phenytoin
c. The patient has never had measles
d. No other family members have a sore throat

393. A 25-year-old female with blonde hair and fair complexion complains of a mole on her upper back. The lesion is 6 mm in diameter, darkly pigmented, and asymmetric, with a very irregular border (see photo). Which of the following is the best next step in management?

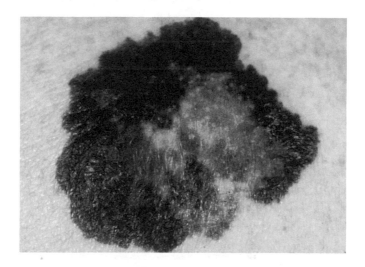

a. Tell the patient to avoid sunlight
b. Follow the lesion for any evidence of growth
c. Obtain metastatic workup
d. Obtain full-thickness excisional biopsy
e. Obtain shave biopsy

394. A 39-year-old male with a prior history of myocardial infarction complains of yellow bumps on his elbows and buttocks. Yellow-colored cutaneous plaques are noted in those areas. The lesions occur in crops and have a surrounding reddish halo. Which of the following is the best next step in evaluation of this patient?

a. Biopsy of skin lesions
b. Lipid profile
c. Uric acid levels
d. Chest x-ray to evaluate for sarcoidosis

395. A 15-year-old girl complains of a low-grade fever, malaise, conjunctivitis, coryza, and cough. After this prodromal phase, a rash of discrete pink macules begins on her face and extends to her hands and feet. She is also noted to have small red spots on her palate. Which of the following is the cause of her rash?

a. Toxic shock syndrome
b. Gonococcal bacteremia
c. Reiter syndrome
d. Rubeola (measles)
e. Rubella (German measles)

396. A 17-year-old girl noted a 2-cm annular pink, scaly lesion on her thigh. In the next 2 weeks she developed several smaller oval pink lesions with a fine collarette of scale. They seem to run in the body folds and mainly involve the trunk, although a few are on the upper arms and thighs. There is no adenopathy and no oral lesions. Which of the following is the most likely diagnosis?

a. Tinea versicolor
b. Psoriasis
c. Lichen planus
d. Pityriasis rosea
e. Secondary syphilis

397. A 45-year-old man with Parkinson's disease has macular areas of erythema and scaling behind the ears and on the scalp, eyebrows, glabella, nasolabial folds, and central chest. Which of the following is the most likely diagnosis?

a. Tinea versicolor
b. Psoriasis
c. Seborrheic dermatitis
d. Atopic dermatitis
e. Dermatophyte infection

398. A 20-year-old white man notes an uneven tan on his upper back and chest. On examination, he has many circular, lighter macules with a barely visible scale that coalesce into larger areas. The best test procedure to establish the diagnosis is which of the following?

a. Punch biopsy
b. Potassium hydroxide (KOH) microscopic examination
c. Dermatophyte test medium (DTM) culture for fungus
d. Serological test for syphilis
e. Tzanck smear

399. A 33-year-old fair-skinned woman has telangiectasias of the cheeks and nose along with red papules and occasional pustules. She also appears to have a conjunctivitis because of dilated scleral vessels. She reports frequent flushing and blushing. Drinking red wine produces a severe flushing of the face. There is a family history of this condition. Which of the following is the most likely diagnosis?

a. Carcinoid syndrome
b. Porphyria cutanea tarda
c. Lupus vulgaris
d. Acne rosacea
e. Seborrheic dermatitis

400. A 46-year-old construction worker is brought to the clinic by his wife because she has noticed an unusual growth on his left ear for the past 8 months (see photo below). The patient explains that except for occasional itching, the lesion does not bother him. On physical exam, you notice an 8-mm pearly papule with a central ulceration and a few small dilated blood vessels on the border. What is the natural course of this lesion if left untreated?

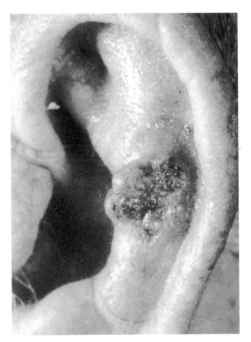

(*Reproduced, with permission, from Kasper DL et al.* Harrison's Principles of Internal Medicine, *16th ed. New York: McGraw-Hill, 2005.*)

a. This is a benign lesion and will not change
b. Local invasion of surrounding tissue
c. Regression over time
d. Local invasion of surrounding tissue and metastasis via lymphatic spread
e. Disseminated infection resulting in septicemia

401. A 25-year-old postal worker presents with a pruritic, nonpainful skin lesion on the dorsum of his hand. It began looking like an insect bite but expanded over several days. On exam, the lesion has a black, necrotic center and is associated with swelling. The patient does not appear to be systemically ill, and vital signs are normal. Which of the following is correct?

a. The lesion is ecthyma gangrenosum, and blood cultures will be positive for *Pseudomonas aeruginosa*
b. A skin biopsy should be performed and Gram stain examined for gram-positive rods
c. The patient has been bitten by *Loxosceles reclusa,* the brown recluse spider
d. The patient has the bubo of plague

402. A 25-year-old who has been living in Washington, DC, presents with a diffuse vesicular rash over his face and trunk. He also has fever. He has no history of chickenpox and has not received the chickenpox vaccine. Which of the following information obtained from history and physical exam suggests that the patient has chickenpox and not smallpox?

a. There are vesicular lesions on the palms and soles
b. All lesions are at the same stage of development
c. The patient experienced high fever several days prior to the rash
d. The rash is more dense over the face than the trunk
e. None of the above

403. A 21-year-old health care worker has been vaccinated for smallpox. After 2 weeks, the site of inoculation fails to heal and the lesion progresses in size with central necrosis and dark eschars. There is little surrounding inflammatory reaction and no pustular lesions. Which of the following is correct?

a. This is a smallpox vaccine complication called vaccinia necrosum; the treatment of choice is vaccinia immune globulin
b. The most likely diagnosis is erythema multiforme
c. The patient is likely to have underlying eczema
d. No evaluation for underlying disease process is necessary

404. A 63-year-old retired farmer presents to the clinic complaining of red scaly spots on his head for the past 9 months. Physical exam is remarkable for several erythematous hyperkeratotic papules and plaques. The lesions are confined to the head and forehead and have poorly defined borders. Which of the following is the most appropriate next step in management of this patient?

a. Punch biopsy of one of the lesions
b. Application of hydrocortisone cream to affected areas and follow-up in 4 weeks
c. Reassurance that this is a benign finding and follow-up in 6 weeks
d. Application of fluocinolone cream to affected areas and follow-up in 4 weeks
e. Application of 5-fluorouracil cream to affected areas and follow-up in 4 weeks

405. A 21-year-old female presents with an annular pruritic rash on her neck. She explains that the rash has been present for the past 3 weeks and that her roommate had a similar rash not too long ago. Physical exam is remarkable for a 21-mm scaling, erythematous plaque with a serpiginous border. Which of the following is the most appropriate initial treatment for this condition?

a. Griseofulvin
b. Oral cephalexin
c. Topical mupirocin ointment
d. Topical ketoconazole
e. Hydrocortisone cream

406. A 34-year-old homosexual male with a history of HIV presents to the clinic complaining of a wheeze and multiple violaceous plaques and nodules on his trunk and extremities. Physical exam of the oral mucosa reveals similar findings on his palate, gingiva, and tongue. Chest x-ray is also significant for pulmonary infiltrates. Which of the following is the most likely etiology for this finding?

a. Proliferation of neoplastic T cells
b. Infection with human herpes virus 6
c. Infection with mycobacterium avium due to decreasing CD4 count
d. Angioproliferative disease caused by infection with human herpes virus 8
e. Disseminated HSV infection

Dermatology

Answers

383. The answer is b. *(Kasper, p 295.)* Isotretinoin has a high potential for teratogenicity and should not be used in women in their childbearing years unless contraception is being practiced. The drug also causes hypertriglyceridemia and drying of mucous membranes. It should be reserved for severe cystic acne. Intralesional triamcinolone is effective for occasional cystic lesions and does not cause systemic side effects. Antimicrobial therapy is of value, in part due to its suppressive effect on *Propionibacterium acnes.* Oral tetracyclines and topical metronidazole are most commonly used.

384. The answer is c. *(Kasper, pp 291–292.)* The rash described is classic for psoriasis, an extremely common chronic inflammatory skin disorder. Its characteristic features include sharply bordered, often round papules or plaques with silver scale, usually located on the knees, elbows, and scalp. Stress, certain medications such as lithium, and skin injury commonly exacerbate the disease. The distribution of the described rash would make contact dermatitis unlikely. Psoriasis is not contagious and is not spread by contact. In the differential of psoriasis is lichen planus (polygonal pruritic purple papules with lacy mucous membrane lesions), pityriasis rosea (herald patch occurs first on trunk in Christmas tree pattern), and dermatophytes (usually less well demarcated, affecting skin, hair, and nails).

385. The answer is c. *(Kasper, pp 999–1001.)* The rash described is most consistent with Rocky Mountain spotted fever, for which a tick is the intermediate vector. Secondary syphilis could present with a macular rash in the same distribution, but the associated symptoms would be atypical. Contact dermatitis would not cause petechial lesions.

386. The answer is c. *(Kasper, p 289.)* Contact dermatitis causes pruritic plaques or vesicles localized to an area of contact. In this case, a bracelet or wristband would be the inciting agent. The dermatitis may have vesicles with weeping lesions. The process is related to direct irritation of the skin from a chemical or physical irritant. It may also be immune-mediated.

marily on extensor surfaces and are associated with elevated triglycerides. Tophaceous gout can result in deposits of monosodium urate, usually in the skin around joints of the hands and feet, that may also be yellow in color. The cutaneous lesions of sarcoidosis are more red-brown in color, appearing as waxy papules, usually on the face. Treatment of hypertriglyceridemia usually results in resolution of lesions. Biopsy of xanthoma would show lipid-containing macrophages, but is usually not necessary for diagnosis.

395. The answer is d. (*Kasper, pp 1148–1153.*) The patient presents with the classic picture of measles. Coryza, conjunctivitis, cough, and fever characterize the measles prodrome. The pathognomonic Koplik spots (pinpoint elevations connected by a network of minute vessels on the soft palate) usually precede onset of the rash by 24 to 48 h and may remain for 2 or 3 days. After the prodrome of 1 to 7 days, the discrete red macules and papules begin behind the ears and spread to the face and trunk, and then distally over the extremities. Toxic shock syndrome produces a diffuse, macular, sunburn-like rash with mucosal hyperemia. Gonococcal bacteremia is more likely to cause nodular skin lesions. In rubella, a maculopapular rash is associated with petechial lesions of the soft palate. Cervical lymphadenopathy is a prominent feature.

396. The answer is d. (*Kasper, pp 292, 979–980.*) The description of this papulosquamous disease is that of a classic case of pityriasis rosea. This disease occurs in about 10% of the population. It is usually seen in young adults on the trunk and proximal extremities. There is a rare inverse form that occurs in the distal extremities and occasionally the face. Pityriasis rosea is usually asymptomatic, although some patients have an early, mild viral prodrome (malaise and low-grade fever), and itching may be significant. Drug eruptions, fungal infections, and secondary syphilis are often confused with this disease. Fungal infections are rarely as widespread and sudden in onset; potassium hydroxide (KOH) preparation will be positive. Syphilis usually is characterized by adenopathy, oral patches, and lesions on the palms and soles (a VDRL test will be strongly positive at this stage). Psoriasis, with its thick, scaly red plaques on extensor surfaces, should not cause confusion. A rare condition called guttate parapsoriasis should be suspected if the rash lasts more than 2 months, since pityriasis rosea usually clears spontaneously in 6 weeks.

397. The answer is c. *(Kasper, pp 291, 1114.)* The patient has the typical areas of involvement of seborrheic dermatitis. This common dermatitis appears to be worse in many neurological diseases. It is also very common and severe in patients with AIDS. In general, symptoms are worse in the winter. *Pityrosporum ovale* appears to play a role in seborrheic dermatitis and dandruff, and the symptoms improve with the use of certain antifungal preparations (e.g., ketoconazole) that decrease this yeast. Mild topical steroids also produce an excellent clinical response.

398. The answer is b. *(Kasper, pp 286–288, 293–294.)* The diagnosis is tinea versicolor, which can be easily confirmed by a KOH microscopic examination. Routine fungal cultures will not grow this yeast. A Wood's light examination will often show a green fluorescence, but it may be negative if the patient has recently showered. A Tzanck smear is used on vesicles to detect herpes infection. A punch biopsy would show the fungus, but is unnecessary, and the fungus might be missed unless special stains are performed.

399. The answer is d. *(Kasper, p 295.)* Rosacea is a common problem in middle-aged, fair-skinned people. Sun damage appears to play an important role. Stress, alcohol, and heat cause flushing. Men may develop rhinophyma (connective tissue overgrowth, particularly of the nose). Low-dose oral tetracycline, erythromycin, and metronidazole control the symptoms. Topical erythromycin and metronidazole also work well.

400. The answer is b. *(Kasper, pp 497–498, 709–711.)* This is a classic description of basal cell carcinoma. Basal cell carcinoma is a malignant neoplasm of the epidermal basal cells that clinically presents as a pearly papule or nodule with a central ulceration, raised borders, and telangiectasias. Basal cell carcinomas are locally invasive and rarely metastasize. A very small percentage of basal cell carcinomas have been shown to metastasize (0.0028 to 0.1%). Invasion of surrounding tissue and metastasis are common characteristics of squamous cell carcinoma. Squamous cell carcinoma is malignant neoplasm of the keratinocytes that is much more aggressive than basal cell carcinoma, grows rapidly, and metastasizes via lymphatic spread. Bacterial infections such as meningococcemia and necrotizing fasciitis could result in septicemia without appropriate treatment.

401. The answer is b. (*Kasper, pp 1279–1283.*) The possibility of cutaneous anthrax in this postal worker is the most important consideration in the era of bioterrorism concern. The lesion described would be characteristic of cutaneous anthrax—beginning as a small papule that is painless and progressing to a black, necrotic lesion over several days. A skin biopsy would show the very characteristic gram-positive rods of anthrax. Cutaneous anthrax has been shown to occur in postal workers who have handled letters that contained anthrax spores, and can also occur in those who handle infected animals or their wool or hides. Ecthyma gangrenosum also produces a black, necrotic skin lesion. These lesions occur in patients who are bacteremic and systemically ill from *P. aeruginosa*. The brown recluse spider's bite can also produce a necrotic ulcer that is black. The bite is painful and usually spreads rapidly. The bubo of plague produces a tender lymphadenitis. It too occurs in a patient who is systemically ill.

402. The answer is e. (*Kasper, 1042–1043, 1284–1285.*) Although there have been no cases of smallpox in the world since 1977, the threat of bioterrorism has forced physicians to be vigilant about the disease's reemergence. It will be important for students and physicians to recognize the distinguishing characteristics of smallpox versus chickenpox. All of the history and physical findings in this case suggest smallpox. Lesions are more likely to occur on palms and soles in smallpox. In chickenpox, lesions are more concentrated on the trunk, whereas in smallpox they are likely to be more concentrated on the face. In smallpox, lesions are characteristically in the same stage of development. In chickenpox, lesions are more superficial, come out in crops, and are in many different stages of development. In smallpox, patients are much more systemically ill, and give a history of fever and prostration prior to the development of the rash. In chickenpox, fever usually occurs at the time of the appearance of the rash.

403. The answer is a. (*Mandell, p 1554.*) The complication of smallpox vaccine described is called vaccinia necrosum or progressive vaccinia. In this disease process, the normal response to vaccination is impaired. The site of the live vaccinia virus inoculation continues to enlarge and fails to heal. As it progresses in size, central necrosis usually occurs. There is little inflammatory reaction. It is usually easily distinguishable from bacterial superinfection. Administration of vaccinia immune globulin is considered the treatment of choice. This immune globulin may be in short supply. Erythema multiforme does occur as an allergic reaction to the vaccine. It is a diffuse erythematous rash with bull's-eye lesions. In patients with eczema, typical vaccinia-type lesions can occur in the areas of active eczema. This process, called eczema vaccinatum, can also be very serious, and patients with eczema should not receive the smallpox vaccine if it can be avoided. In a patient with vaccinia necrosum, it is important to consider underlying immunodeficiency disease such as HIV or other immunodeficiency disease.

404. The answer is e. *(Kasper, pp 497–498. Wolff, pp 262–264.)* Actinic keratoses are premalignant lesions of the skin with the potential to degenerate into squamous cell carcinoma. If left untreated, up to 20% of these lesions can become malignant. Diagnosis is usually made clinically through history and physical examination of the skin. These lesions often present as erythematous hyperkeratotic papules or plaques on sun-exposed areas. They have poorly defined borders and are easier to feel because of their scaly texture. Treatment can be done with either cryotherapy (liquid nitrogen) or application of topical 5-fluorouracil. Cryotherapy is the preferred method when there are a few lesions. However, when there are many lesions with poorly defined borders, 5-fluorouracil may be used. Topical corticosteroids such as hydrocortisone or fluocinolone would not be used for treatment of actinic keratoses.

405. The answer is d. *(Kasper, pp 1191–1192.)* Tinea corporis (ringworm) is a dermatophyte that causes a superficial infection of the skin. Tinea corporis clinically presents as an erythematous scaly plaque with a central clearing and serpiginous border. It is usually acquired through contact with an infected individual or animal. Initial treatment involves application of topical antifungals such as ketoconazole, clotrimazole, miconazole, toconazole, econazole, naftifine, terbinafine, or ciclopirox olamine cream. A more severe infection that is unresponsive to topical therapy, or one involving the scalp, nails, or bearded area, should be treated systematically with oral griseofluvin, itraconazole, or terbinafine. Cephalexin and mupirocin are antibacterial agents used for superficial infections of the skin caused by *Staphylococcus aureus* such as folliculitis or impetigo. Hydrocortisone is a weak corticosteroid that can actually exacerbate a fungal infection.

406. The answer is d. *(Kasper, p 1098. Wolff, pp 536–540.)* This patient has Kaposi's sarcoma (KS). In HIV-infected individuals KS is associated with human herpes virus 8 (HHV-8). KS lesions are derived from the proliferation of endothelial cells in blood/lymphatic microvasculature. They present as violaceous patches, plaques, and/or nodules on the skin, mucosa, and/or viscera. The pulmonary infiltrates observed on the chest x-ray for this patient are the result of visceral KS affecting the lungs. Proliferation of neoplastic T cells is seen in cutaneous T cell lymphomas such as mycosis fungoides. Human herpes virus 6 (HHV-6) is the cause of exanthema subitum (roseola) in children. It consists of 2- to 3-mm pink macules and papules on the trunk following a fever. Mycobacterium avium causes pulmonary infection in HIV patients with a CD4 count <50/μL. Immunodeficient patients or patients with HIV who are infected with HSV can present with the disseminated form of the disease. However, these lesions consist of a vesicular rash that is different from the violaceous lesions observed in KS.

General Medicine and Prevention

Questions

DIRECTIONS: Each item below contains a question followed by suggested responses. Select the **one best** response to each question.

407. A 53-year-old female presents to the emergency room with a minor injury and is found to have a blood pressure of 150/102, possibly elevated due to pain. On follow-up at your office, her BP on two occasions is 142/94 despite good dietary habits and reasonable exercise. Her history and physical are essentially normal except that she has had a hysterectomy. Basic lab evaluation reveals no significant abnormalities. Based on recent recommendations of the JNC 7 (The Seventh Report of the Joint National Committee on Prevention, Detection, Evaluation, and Treatment of High Blood Pressure) which of the following is accurate information to give her?

a. At age >50, high diastolic BP becomes a more important cardiovascular risk factor than high systolic
b. The new classification of prehypertension fits her latest BP readings; continue close follow-up
c. Thiazide diuretics are being emphasized as the initial antihypertensive for most and would be a good choice for her
d. Initiating therapy with two antihypertensives would be preferred based on her current BP
e. Estrogen-replacement therapy would be helpful in delaying her need for antihypertensives

408. A patient with type 2 diabetes mellitus is found to have a blood pressure of 152/98. She has never had any ophthalmologic, cardiovascular, or renal complications of diabetes or hypertension. Which of the following is the currently recommended goal for blood pressure control in this case?

a. Less than 160/90
b. Less than 145/95
c. Less than 140/90
d. Less than 130/80
e. Less than 120/70

409. A 60-year-old white male just moved to town and needs to establish care for coronary artery disease, given the fact that he had a "heart attack" last year. Preferring a "natural" approach, he has been very conscientious about low-fat, low-cholesterol eating habits and a significant exercise program, but gradually eliminated a number of prescription medications (he does not recall their names) that he was on at the time of hospital discharge. Past history is negative for hypertension, diabetes, or smoking. The lipid profile you obtain shows the following:

Total cholesterol: 198 mg/dL
Triglycerides: 160 mg/dL
HDL: 42
LDL (calculated): 124

Which of the following recommendations would most optimally treat his lipid status?

a. Continue current dietary efforts and exercise
b. Add an HMG-CoA reductase inhibitor (statin drug)
c. Add a fibric acid derivative such as gemfibrozil
d. Review previous medications and resume an angiotensin-converting enzyme inhibitor

410. A 60-year-old male had an anterior myocardial infarction 3 months ago. He currently is asymptomatic and has normal vital signs and a normal physical exam. He is on an antiplatelet agent and an ACE inhibitor. What other category of medication would typically be prescribed for secondary prevention of myocardial infarction?

a. Alpha blocker
b. Beta blocker
c. Calcium channel blocker
d. Nitrates

411. A 50-year-old white male who comes for general checkup is a healthy nonsmoker, free of hypertension, diabetes, or cardiac disease. However, his 53-year-old brother had coronary artery bypass surgery this year. You order a fasting lipid profile and are able to calculate his coronary heart disease 10-year risk as 6%. Which of the following is the currently recommended LDL target level for this patient?

a. Less than 160 mg/dL
b. Less than 130 mg/dL
c. Less than 100 mg/dL
d. Less than 70 mg/dL

412. A 58-year-old male has a history of hypertension and asks about reducing his risk for myocardial infarction. A lipid profile is obtained that shows a low HDL cholesterol of 32 mg/dL. An important recommendation in attempting to raise the HDL would be:

a. Aspirin, one tablet each day
b. Dehydroepiandrosterone (DHEA)
c. Vitamin E, 400 U each day
d. Folic acid plus pyridoxine (vitamin B$_6$)
e. Exercise

413. A 32-year-old diabetic female who takes an estrogen-containing oral contraceptive and drinks three beers per day is found to have a triglyceride level greater than 1000 mg/dL. She is at most risk for which of the following complications?

a. Acute pancreatitis
b. Sudden cardiac death
c. Acute peripheral arterial occlusion
d. Acute renal insufficiency
e. Myositis

414. A 28-year-old, otherwise healthy white female on no medications presents to the ER with chest pressure, dizziness, numbness in both hands, and feeling of impending doom that began while walking in the mall. Physical exam reveals no specific abnormalities. The most appropriate direction to take in the management plan would be which of the following?

a. Exercise stress testing
b. Echocardiography
c. Empiric proton pump inhibitor therapy
d. Reassurance plus alprazolam and/or antidepressant therapy
e. Chest CT scan with consideration of IV heparin

415. A 45-year-old, generally healthy female on no medications comes to your office with a 10-day history of nasal congestion, sore throat, dry cough, and initial low-grade fever, all of which were nearly resolved. However, over the past 24 to 48 h she has developed a sharp chest pain, worse with deep inspiration or cough, but no dyspnea. Due to the severity of the pain, the nurse had obtained an ECG, which showed diffuse ST elevation. On physical exam, you expect the most likely finding to be which of the following?

a. A loud pulmonic component of S_2
b. An S_3 gallop
c. A pericardial friction rub
d. Bilateral basilar rales
e. Elevated blood pressure >160/100

416. A 25-year-old male PhD candidate recently traveled to Central America for 1 month to gain further information for his dissertation regarding the socioeconomics of that region. While there, he took ciprofloxacin twice a day for 5 days for diarrhea. However, over the 2 to 3 weeks since coming home, he has continued to have occasional loose stools plus vague abdominal discomfort and bloating. There has been no rectal bleeding. Which of the following therapies is most likely to relieve this traveler's diarrhea?

a. Ciprofloxacin (repeat course)
b. Doxycycline
c. Metronidazole
d. Trimethoprim-sulfa (Bactrim DS)
e. Oral glucose-electrolyte solution

417. A 25-year-old asymptomatic HIV-positive male with CD4+ cell count of 525 comes to you for travel advice and immunizations prior to a trip to Indonesia. Which of the following is an inappropriate recommendation?

a. Give tetanus-diphtheria booster if not up-to-date
b. Give oral polio booster if not up-to-date
c. Start hepatitis B immunization series if never received
d. Give pneumococcal vaccine if never received
e. Give second MMR if only one dose previously received
f. Give malaria prophylaxis

418. In August you saw a debilitated 80-year-old female who required nursing home placement. She had had no immunizations for many years except for a pneumococcal vaccine 3 years ago when discharged from the hospital after a stay for pneumonia. Appropriate admission orders to the nursing home in August included which of the following?

a. Flu shot
b. *Haemophilus influenzae* B immunization
c. Hepatitis B immunization series
d. Pneumococcal revaccination
e. Tetanus-diphtheria toxoid booster

419. An asymptomatic 50-year-old man who has smoked one pack of cigarettes per day for 30 years comes to you for a general checkup and wants "the works" for cancer screening. In fact, he hands you a list of tests he desires. Which test is inappropriate based on American Cancer Society guidelines?

a. Chest x-ray
b. Digital rectal exam
c. Flexible sigmoidoscopy
d. Prostate-specific antigen (PSA) blood test
e. Skin exam

420. An asymptomatic 35-year-old female comes to you for routine exam. She has no unusual family history of breast cancer. Based on American Cancer Society guidelines for early detection of breast cancer, this patient at standard risk should be advised to do which of the following?

a. Perform breast self-examination monthly
b. Obtain physician-performed breast examination yearly
c. Begin yearly mammograms
d. Obtain genetic testing via blood work as a baseline
e. Wait until age 40 to begin cancer screening

421. On presentation for yearly exam, a healthy, non–sexually active, postmenopausal 60-year-old female gives a history of having had normal yearly mammograms and normal yearly Pap smears over the past 10 years, but has never had an endometrial tissue sample or any screening test for ovarian cancer. The most clearly indicated cancer screening evaluation on today's visit is which of the following?

a. Bilateral mammogram
b. Pap smear
c. Endometrial tissue sample
d. CA 125 blood test
e. CEA level

422. You have been asked to perform a preoperative consultation on a 66-year-old male who will be undergoing transurethral resection of the prostate for urinary retention. Of the following findings, which you detect by history, physical, ECG, and lab, which is of most concern in predicting a cardiac complication in this patient undergoing noncardiac surgery?

a. Age over 65
b. Current cigarette use at one pack per day
c. Serum creatinine 2.2 mg/dL
d. History of three alcoholic drinks/day with ALT (SGOT) 60 mg/dL
e. ECG (and subsequent cardiac monitoring) with right bundle branch block and 5 PVCs/minute
f. The nature of the surgery itself (on the high-risk list)

423. A 42-year-old male is persuaded by his wife to come to you for general checkup. She hints of concern about alcohol use. Therefore, you ask the CAGE questions as an initial screen. These include which of the following?

a. Concern expressed by family
b. Previous Alcoholics Anonymous contact
c. Alcohol intake greater than two drinks per 24 h
d. Gastrointestinal symptoms
e. Use of an eye-opener
f. Presence of excess extremity shakiness

424. A 78-year-old female comes to your office with symptoms of insomnia nearly every day, fatigue, weight loss of over 5% of body weight over the past month, loss of interest in most activities, and diminished ability to concentrate. Although further testing may be necessary, based on this history the most likely approach to therapy will involve which of the following?

a. Antidepressant
b. Cholinesterase inhibitor such as donepezil
c. Iron supplement
d. Prednisone
e. Thyroid supplement

425. A 65-year-old female was hospitalized for pulmonary embolus and eventually discharged on warfarin (Coumadin) with a therapeutic INR. During the next 2 weeks as an outpatient, she was started back on her previous ACE inhibitor antihypertensive, given temazepam for insomnia, treated with ciprofloxacin for a urinary tract infection, started on over-the-counter famotidine (Pepcid) for GI symptoms, and told to stop the OTC naproxen she was taking. Follow-up INR was too high, most likely due to which of the following?

a. ACE inhibitor therapy
b. Temazepam
c. Ciprofloxacin
d. Famotidine (Pepcid)
e. Naproxen discontinuation

426. A 20-year-old college basketball player is brought to the university urgent care clinic after developing chest pain and palpitations during practice, but no dyspnea or tachypnea. There is no unusual family history of cardiac diseases, and social history is negative for alcohol or drug use. Cardiac auscultation is unremarkable, and ECG shows only occasional PVCs. Which of the following is the most appropriate next step in evaluation and/or management?

a. Obtain urine drug screen
b. Arrange treadmill stress test
c. Obtain Doppler ultrasound of deep veins of lower legs
d. Institute cardioselective beta blocker therapy
e. Institute respiratory therapy for this form of exercise-induced bronchospasm

427. A 92-year-old woman with type 2 diabetes mellitus has developed cellulitis and gangrene of her left foot. She requires a lifesaving amputation, but refuses to give consent for the surgery. She has been ambulatory in her nursing home but states that she would be so dependent after surgery that life would not be worth living for her. She has no living relatives; she enjoys walks and gardening. She is competent and of clear mind. Which of the following is the most appropriate course of action?

a. Perform emergency surgery
b. Consult a psychiatrist
c. Request permission for surgery from a friend of the patient
d. Follow the patient's wishes

428. A 20-year-old complains of diarrhea, burning of the throat, and difficulty swallowing over 2 months. On exam, he has mild jaundice and transverse white striae of the fingernails. There is also evidence for peripheral neuropathy. Which of the following is the best diagnostic study in this case?

a. Liver biopsy
b. Arsenic level
c. Antinuclear antibody
d. Endoscopy (EGD)
e. TSH plus free T_4

429. A young boy believes he was bitten by a spider while playing in his attic. Severe pain develops at the site of the bite after several hours. Bullae and erythema develop around the bite, and some skin necrosis becomes apparent. The boy is afebrile without evidence of toxicity. This is most likely which of the following?

a. A black widow (*Latrodectus mactans*) spider bite, with local wound care the initial therapy
b. A black widow (*Latrodectus mactans*) spider bite, with antivenin indicated as soon as possible
c. A brown recluse (*Loxosceles* sp.) spider bite, with local wound care the initial therapy
d. A brown recluse (*Loxosceles* sp.) spider bite, with early but rapidly progressing streptococcal necrotizing fasciitis

430. A 70-year-old male with unresectable carcinoma of the lung metasta-tic to liver and bone has developed progressive weight loss, anorexia, and shortness of breath. The patient has executed a valid living will that pro-hibits the use of feeding tube in the setting of terminal illness. The patient becomes lethargic and stops eating altogether. The patient's wife of 30 years insists on enteral feeding for her husband. Since he has become unable to take in adequate nutrition, which of the following is the most appropriate course of action?

a. Respect the wife's wishes as a reliable surrogate decision maker
b. Resist the placement of a feeding tube in accordance with the living will
c. Call a family conference to get broad input from others
d. Place a feeding tube until such time as the matter can be discussed with the patient

431. After being stung by a yellow jacket, a 14-year-old develops the sud-den onset of hoarseness and shortness of breath. An urticarial rash is noted. Which of the following is the most important first step in treatment?

a. An antihistamine
b. Epinephrine
c. Venom immunotherapy
d. Corticosteroids
e. Removal of the stinger

432. A 40-year-old male is found to have a uric acid level of 9 mg/dL on a comprehensive blood chemistry profile. The patient has never had gouty arthritis, renal disease, or kidney stones. The patient has no evidence on history or physical exam of underlying chronic or malignant disease. The approach to this patient is best stated by which of the following?

a. The risk of urolithiasis requires the institution of prophylactic therapy such as allopurinol
b. Asymptomatic hyperuricemia is associated with an increased risk of gouty arthritis, but benefits of prophylaxis do not outweigh risks in this patient
c. Further investigation beyond history and physical is needed to assess for lym-phoproliferative disease
d. Hyperuricemia is associated with cardiovascular disease; its treatment will lower this risk

433. A 38-year-old obese female with history of chronic venous insufficiency and peripheral edema was admitted to the hospital the previous night for cellulitis involving both lower legs. She has had recurrent such episodes, treated successfully in the past with various antibiotics, including cefazolin, nafcillin, ampicillin/sulbactam, and even levofloxacin. Intravenous levofloxacin was again chosen due to the perceived ease in transitioning to a once-daily oral outpatient dose. Past history is otherwise significant only for hypertension, which is being treated at home with HCTZ 25 mg, lisinopril 40 mg, and atenolol 100 mg, all once each morning. Admission BP was 144/92 and the orders were written to continue each of these antihypertensives at one tablet po qd. The only other in-hospital medication is daily prophylactic enoxaparin. As you round at 6 P.M. on the day following admission, the nurse contacts you emergently stating that she has just finished giving evening meds and the patient's BP is unexpectedly 90/50. There is no chest pain, dyspnea, or tachypnea. Which of the following etiologies for hypotension is most likely?

a. An allergic reaction to either the antibiotic or one of the antihypertensives
b. A vasovagal reaction secondary to pain
c. Hypovolemia due to the cellulitis
d. The new onset of diabetic ketoacidosis
e. Acute pulmonary embolism
f. Medication error
g. Herbal product use by the patient while in the hospital

434. A 44-year-old Hispanic female comes to clinic for a general checkup due to concern about a family history of diabetes and high blood pressure. Her height is 62 in, weight 50 kg (110 lb), blood pressure 138/88. Lab evaluation reveals fasting glucose of 120 mg/dL. Lipid profile shows total cholesterol 240 mg/dL, HDL 38 mg/dL, and triglycerides 420 mg/dL; LDL cannot be calculated. She does not smoke, use alcohol, or take any medications. Which of the following is correct regarding the identification of the metabolic syndrome in this patient?

a. This syndrome is not present in this case due to the absence of abdominal obesity
b. This is not present because the blood pressure is not sufficiently elevated to be a risk factor
c. This syndrome is not present because the glucose is not sufficiently elevated to be a risk factor
d. This syndrome is present based on the risk factors given
e. This syndrome cannot be identified until the LDL is determined
f. This syndrome cannot be identified until the presence of hyperuricemia is established

DIRECTIONS: Each group of questions below consists of lettered options followed by a set of numbered items. For each numbered item, select the **one** lettered option with which it is **most** closely associated. Each lettered option may be used once, more than once, or not at all.

Questions 435–437

The initial choice of an antihypertensive or the addition of further agent(s) to the regimen may depend on concomitant factors. For each of the cases below, indicate the medication choice that would give the best additional benefit after blood pressure control.

a. Alpha blocker
b. Beta blocker
c. Calcium channel blocker
d. Angiotensin-converting enzyme inhibitor
e. Centrally acting agent
f. Diuretic

435. A 67-year-old African-American male complains of tendency toward urinary retention. Digital rectal exam reveals enlarged prostate.

436. An obese 54-year-old white female has hemoglobin A_{1C} of 9.5 and elevated urine microalbumin.

437. A 62-year-old female still experiences occasional migraine headaches and has now begun having a tremor involving both hands.

Questions 438–440

The choice of an antihypertensive agent may involve trying to avoid an adverse effect on a comorbid condition. For each of the patients with known hypertension below, indicate the medication choice that needs to be avoided above all others.

a. Angiotensin-converting enzyme inhibitor
b. Beta blocker, noncardioselective
c. Calcium channel blocker
d. Diuretic
e. Hydralazine

438. A 40-year-old white male has three episodes over the past two years of debilitating acute arthritis involving various ankle and foot joints.

439. A 70-year-old male with COPD quit smoking 5 years ago, but is now beginning to experience cramps in his calf muscles upon walking one block. Diminished popliteal and pedal pulses are noted on exam.

440. A 24-year-old single female has delayed seeing a doctor over the past 3 months due to lack of insurance; she has experienced amenorrhea and nausea.

Questions 441–444

For each patient below with latent tuberculosis infection with negative chest x-ray, select the best course of action.

a. Begin three- to four-drug antituberculosis regimen
b. Begin two-drug antituberculosis regimen
c. Begin isoniazid alone
d. No treatment indicated
e. Repeat PPD in 2 weeks

441. An HIV-positive patient has 5-mm PPD.

442. A 70-year-old new patient at a nursing home has 8-mm PPD.

443. A 40-year-old has 10-mm PPD; there is no underlying illness; this was the first time it was done.

444. A 60-year-old woman had negative PPD 1 year ago; she now has 12-mm PPD on annual screening.

General Medicine and Prevention

Answers

407. The answer is c. (*JNC 7 Express, p xiii.*) A key point in the JNC 7 is that a thiazide diuretic should be used in most patients with uncomplicated hypertension when diet and lifestyle modifications are not sufficient. Other major points include (1) systolic BP > 140 is a more important cardiovascular risk factor than diastolic BP in persons over age 50; (2) individuals normotensive at age 55 still have a 90% lifetime risk of developing hypertension, and CVD risk doubles, beginning at 115/75, for each rise in BP of 20/10; (3) a new category of prehypertension has been designated with systolic BP 120 to 139 or diastolic BP 80 to 89, with emphasis on healthy diet and lifestyle modifications; (4) most patients will require two or more antihypertensives to achieve goal BP, which is <140/90 except in diabetes or renal disease; (5) if BP > 20/10 above goal is present at the outset, consider initiating therapy with two agents. Estrogen-replacement plays no beneficial cardiovascular role here.

408. The answer is d. (*JNC 7 Express, pp 7, 15. Kasper, p 1479.*) Goals for blood pressure control and lipid levels are typically more stringent in the diabetic compared to the nondiabetic. The previously recommended goal blood pressure of <130/85 has been shifted down to <130/80. The same is true for those with renal disease.

409. The answer is b. (*NCEP ATP III, pp 2–4, 7–9, 12–14. Kasper, p 1430–1431, 2295–2296.*) The National Cholesterol Education Program Adult Treatment Panel III recommendations include lowering the LDL cholesterol to <100 mg/dL in those with known coronary heart disease (secondary prevention). The 2004 update to these guidelines adds an optional goal of LDL < 70 mg/dL in very high risk patients. In this case, with dietary efforts and exercise already well-established and unlikely to reduce LDL further, a statin drug is indicated. These typically lower LDL by 20 to 50%. Gemfibrozil is used primarily for hypertriglyceridemia. ACE inhibitors have no significant effect on lipids.

410. The answer is b. (*Kasper, pp 1440–1441, 1459, 1477.*) Beta blockers are documented to lower the risk of myocardial reinfarction, whereas calcium channel blockers may increase the risk. Alpha blockers have been associated with an increased risk of congestive heart failure. ACE inhibitors are beneficial in this setting, and the data is accumulating that angiotensin II receptor blockers are as well. Despite their decades-long use in the treatment of coronary artery disease, such as for angina, nitrates are not indicated for secondary prevention of infarction.

411. The answer is b. (*NCEP ATP III, pp 2–5. Kasper, p 1430–1431.*) The National Cholesterol Education Program Adult Treatment Panel III primary prevention guidelines include lowering the LDL to <160 mg/dL if the patient is free of coronary heart disease and with zero or one risk factor. Less than 130 mg/dL is recommended if free of coronary heart disease and with two or more risk factors. These risk factors include cigarette smoking, hypertension (BP 140/90 or greater, or an antihypertensive medication), low HDL cholesterol (<40 mg/dL), family history of premature coronary heart disease (CHD in first-degree male relative <55 years or in female <65 years old), and age (men 45 years old or greater; women 55 or greater). The goal is <100 mg/dL in the presence of known coronary heart disease or coronary heart disease equivalents such as diabetes or calculated CHD 10-year risk of >20%. In this example, although the patient is healthy, he has two risk factors by virtue of being male age 45 years or older, plus family history of early coronary heart disease, but the CHD 10-year risk is low. Therefore the goal is <130. If specific BP and lipid numbers had been given in the question and his CHD 10-year risk had calculated to be in the 10 to 20% range (i.e., moderately high risk), the new 2004 ATP III update adds a more aggressive optional goal of <100.

412. The answer is e. (*Kasper, pp 1431–1432, 2295. NCEP ATP III, pp 19–20.*) Within this group of choices, only exercise has been shown to raise HDL. Among current lipid-lowering medications, nicotinic acid has the most potent HDL-increasing effect at 15 to 35%, followed by fibric acids and then statins. Alcohol also increases the HDL level (HDL2 and HDL3 subfractions), thereby imparting some cardioprotective effect, but at the risk of cardiomyopathy, sudden death, hemorrhagic stroke, and other non-cardiovascular problems among heavy drinkers. The cardiovascular system may benefit from aspirin via antiplatelet effects and folic acid/pyridoxine via lowering high homocysteine levels; after initial enthusiasm for vitamin E, more recent studies have not shown consistent cardiovascular benefit from antioxidant vitamins. None of these raise HDL. DHEA lowers HDL.

413. The answer is a. (*Kasper, pp 1896, 2294–2295.*) Hypertriglyceridemia, which is enhanced by poorly controlled diabetes, estrogen, and alcohol, predisposes to pancreatitis.

414. The answer is d. (*Kasper, pp 2547–2549.*) Although other possibilities need to be considered and possibly evaluated, the patient's age and symptoms are consistent with panic disorder. The diagnostic criteria for panic attack are a discrete period of intense fear or discomfort, in which four or more of the following symptoms develop abruptly and reach a peak within 10 min: palpitations, pounding heart, or accelerated heart rate; sweating; trembling or shaking; sensations of shortness of breath or smothering; feeling of choking; chest pain or discomfort; nausea or abdominal distress; feeling dizzy, unsteady, lightheaded, or faint; derealization or depersonalization; fear of losing control or going crazy; fear of dying; paresthesias; chills or hot flushes. Patient education/awareness is fundamentally important. Drug therapy may consist of antidepressants and/or the benzodiazepine alprazolam. The other answers allude to diagnoses of angina or other heart disease, gastroesophageal reflux, or pulmonary embolus. Angina would be unlikely in such a young female; GERD also more likely in an older person and typically at night upon lying down; PE not likely with normal exam, including absence of tachypnea.

415. The answer is c. (*Kasper, pp 1414–1415.*) This history and ECG suggest acute postviral pericarditis, in which the most likely confirmatory physical finding of those listed would be the pericardial friction rub. This may be transitory and may best be heard in expiration with patient upright or leaning forward. A loud S_2 might be heard with a pulmonary embolus, an S_3 gallop with CHF, and bibasilar rales with CHF or possibly pneumonia.

416. The answer is c. (*Kasper, pp 754–759, 1248–1250.*) *Giardia lamblia* gives the subacute to chronic picture as described in this patient and responds to metronidazole therapy. It is contracted by ingesting contaminated food or water, with the classic zoonotic reservoirs being the freshwater streams of the northern United States and also the water supplies in Russia and developing countries. Bacterial pathogens such as *Campylobacter jejuni*, enterotoxigenic *E. coli*, *Salmonella*, and *Shigella* usually cause acute diarrhea, often bloody. They usually respond to fluoroquinolones or azithromycin. Oral glucose-electrolyte solution rehydration is the mainstay of *Vibrio cholerae* therapy. Hydration rather than antibiotics is also the key for enterohemorrhagic *E. coli*.

417. The answer is b. (*Kasper, pp 721–722, 729.*) The usual immunizations may be given to an HIV-infected person, preferably as early in the course as possible, except for oral polio vaccine (and varicella). OPV yields an unacceptably high risk of live virus proliferation and paralytic polio. Immunocompromised persons and their household contacts should receive inactivated poliovirus vaccine (IPV), not OPV.

418. The answer is e. (*Kasper, pp 717–718, 720.*) A Td (adult tetanus-diphtheria booster) should be given every 10 years. A flu shot should be given in this age group, but at the appropriate time in the fall. There is no recommendation to give the *Haemophilus* immunization in adults. This patient is not in one of the high-risk categories for hepatitis B (including health care workers, hemodialysis patients, routine recipients of clotting factors, travelers to endemic areas, persons at elevated risk for sexually transmitted diseases, injection drug users, those in institutions for the mentally retarded, and household contacts of hepatitis B carriers) and therefore has no specific indication to receive this series. The pneumococcal vaccine may be given again to higher-risk individuals at least 5 years after the original.

419. The answer is a. (*Kasper, pp 445–447, 509, 529, 544.*) Neither the chest x-ray nor any other test has proven to be an effective screen for lung cancer (although spiral chest CT shows some promise). The digital rectal exam aids in screening for rectal and prostate cancer. Other options regarding colorectal cancer are flexible sigmoidoscopy every 5 years, colonoscopy every 10 years, or double-contrast barium enema every 5 to 10 years. PSA levels, though somewhat controversial, play a role in prostate cancer screening. The physical exam remains important (e.g., in detection of testicular and skin cancers), although definitive evidence regarding screening is sparse.

420. The answer is a. *(Kasper, pp 445–446, 519.)* For early detection of breast cancer, the American Cancer Society recommends breast self-examination monthly starting at age 20; breast physical examination every 3 years from ages 20 to 40, then yearly; and mammography every year beginning at age 40. Other organizations advise mammography every 1 to 2 years from ages 40 to 50, then yearly, possibly stopping at age 70 or 75.

421. The answer is a. *(Kasper, pp 445–446, 519, 554, 557.)* Breast cancer is the most common of women's cancers. Mammography is still recommended yearly from age 50 upward (and every 1 to 2 years from ages 40 to 50, depending on the organization, some of which also conclude exams at age 70 or 75). Pap smears to screen for cervical cancer may be performed yearly, but after three consecutive normal exams this may be done less frequently. Endometrial tissue samples for uterine cancer become important at menopause if at high risk. There is no true screening test for ovarian cancer at present. CEA levels are not recommended as a colon cancer screen.

422. The answer is c. *(Kasper, pp 39–41.)* The original standard for the measurement of cardiac risk in the setting of noncardiac surgery was the Goldman index. The American Heart Association and American College of Cardiology also have guidelines. More recently, the revised cardiac risk index of Lee has gained preference as more accurate. Its six predictive factors for post-op cardiac complications are high-risk type of surgery (intraperitoneal, intrathoracic, or suprainguinal vascular), ischemic heart disease, history of congestive heart failure, history of symptomatic cerebrovascular disease, insulin therapy for diabetes, and pre-op serum creatinine > 2.0 mg/dL. Only the last of these applies to this case.

423. The answer is e. *(Kasper, p 1810.)* The CAGE screening tool for alcoholism consists of asking about alcohol-related trouble: cutting down, being annoyed by criticisms, guilt, and use of an eye-opener (i.e., alcohol consumption upon arising).

424. The answer is a. *(Kasper, pp 2553–2554.)* Depression is commonly encountered in the outpatient setting and probably underlies the chief complaint of fatigue more than any other cause. Among the criteria for diagnosis are the presence during the same 2-week period of five or more of nine specific symptoms. Five of these are mentioned in the question; the other four are depressed mood, psychomotor agitation or retardation, feelings of worthlessness, and recurrent thoughts of death (or suicidal ideation). Thus psychotherapy and antidepressant medication would be the basic treatment.

425. The answer is c. *(Kasper, p 692.)* Many medications can potentiate warfarin (Coumadin), including the fluoroquinolone ciprofloxacin and various other broad-spectrum antibiotics. The other choices do not. Nonsteroidal anti-inflammatory drugs may occasionally enhance warfarin's effect, so discontinuing naproxen, if anything, should lower the INR. If the H_2 blocker cimetidine or the proton pump inhibitor omeprazole had been used for gastric acid reduction in this case, either of these can potentiate warfarin and increase the INR. Of interest is that one other increasingly seen potentiator of warfarin is the over-the-counter herbal product ginkgo biloba.

426. The answer is a. *(Kasper, pp 2570–2571.)* The question of cocaine use must be raised in virtually all young adults with cardiovascular symptoms, despite a professed negative history. Therefore, a urine drug screen should be obtained early on. If this is negative, the patient might well need further cardiac evaluation, such as echocardiogram, ambulatory cardiac monitoring, and/or stress test.

427. The answer is d. *(Kasper, p 4.)* The principle of autonomy is an overriding issue in this patient, who is competent to make her own decisions about surgery. Consulting a psychiatrist would be inappropriate unless there is some reason to believe the patient is not competent. No such concern is present in this description of the patient. Since the patient is competent, no friend or relative can give permission for the procedure.

428. The answer is b. *(Kasper, p 2577.)* Although there is no clue to exposure (pesticides, herbicides; wood preservatives; smelting and microelectronics by-products; contamination of deep water wells; folk remedies), the clinical picture is characteristic of arsenic poisoning. Manifestations of toxicity are varied but include irritation of the GI tract, resulting in the symptoms described. Arsenic combines with the globin chain of hemoglobin to produce hemolysis. The white transverse lines of the fingernails, called Aldrich-Mees lines, are a manifestation of chronic arsenic poisoning.

429. The answer is c. *(Kasper, pp 2603–2604.)* Bites from *Loxosceles* spiders (including the brown recluse) may cause necrosis of tissue at the site of the bite. The cause of the local reaction is not well understood but is thought to involve complement-mediated tissue damage. Dapsone, steroids, and antivenin have all been used in treatment, but no therapy is of proven value. The bite of the black widow spider causes neurologic signs and abdominal pain but does not result in soft tissue damage. Without fever and toxicity, the skin signs described are not likely to be secondary to bacterial infection.

430. The answer is b. *(Kasper, pp 4, 56–57.)* The patient's autonomy as directed by the living will must be respected. This autonomy is not transferred to a surrogate decision maker, even one who is very credible. A family conference in this case would not change the overriding issue—that a valid living will is in effect.

431. The answer is b. *(Kasper, p 2605.)* The administration of epinephrine is the best treatment in the acute setting. Epinephrine provides both α- and β-adrenergic effects. Antihistamines and corticosteroids are frequently given as well, although they have little immediate effect. The patient should be offered venom immunotherapy after recovery from the systemic reaction. Removal without compression of an insect stinger is worthwhile, but not the primary concern.

432. The answer is b. *(Kasper, pp 2309–2311.)* Asymptomatic hyperuricemia does increase the risk of acute gouty arthritis, but most hyperuricemic individuals never have an episode. The cost of lifelong prophylaxis is high, as is the risk of an adverse reaction to a drug like allopurinol, such that the more conservative approach is favored of treating an acute attack when it occurs. Prophylactic therapy would be reserved for patients with repeated acute attacks. Likewise the risk of urolithiasis is sufficiently low that prophylaxis is not necessary until the development of a stone. Structural kidney damage is not identifiable before a first gouty attack. Hyperuricemia is associated with but not a cause of arteriosclerotic disease and there is no proven cardiovascular benefit to reducing the uric acid level. However, an elevated uric level may be a clue to look for diabetes, hypertension, and/or hyperlipidemia. In patients with lymphoproliferative disease, prophylaxis for the prevention of renal impairment is recommended, especially in the face of chemotherapy.

433. The answer is f. (*Kasper, pp 4–5.*) The concept being advanced here is medication error. A new emphasis is being placed on reducing all medical errors, including those related to misreading of handwriting, which might include avoidance of certain abbreviations or use of an electronic medical record. In this case the pharmacist and/or nurse mistook the medication orders for one tablet po qd (once a day) for one tablet po qid (four times a day), such that the patient had received three doses of each antihypertensive by 6 P.M. There is no particular clue to the other listed answers. For example, an allergic reaction would seem unlikely with medications previously well tolerated; there are no symptoms or signs of acute pulmonary embolism, and a prophylactic anticoagulant is in use. The use by the patient within the hospital of substances from outside, unknown to the medical staff, is a valid consideration. Related to effect on blood pressure, the main herbal product adverse effect is an elevated BP from those containing ephedrine.

434. The answer is d. (*NCEP ATP III, pp 15–17. Kasper, pp 1431–1432, 2311.*) The metabolic syndrome represents a cluster of metabolic risk factors for coronary heart disease, closely linked to insulin resistance. It can be identified when any three of the following five items are present: abdominal obesity [waist circumference in women >88 cm (>35 in) or in men >102 cm (40 in)]; hypertriglyceridemia (>150 mg/dL); low HDL (<50 mg/dL in women or <40 in men); blood pressure greater than or equal to 130/85; and fasting glucose > 110 mg/dL. In this case, four risk factors are present, all except abdominal obesity. In addition, hyperinsulinemia decreases the renal excretion of uric acid, resulting in hyperuricemia, although this finding is not part of the metabolic syndrome definition.

435–437. The answers are 435-a, 436-d, 437-b. (*JNC 7 Express, pp 15–19. Kasper, pp 545, 1472–1479.*) Alpha blockers such as terazosin or doxazosin improve urinary outflow and might benefit a male with benign prostatic hypertrophy with urinary retention when used as an addition to another antihypertensive; use of this class as a single agent has been discouraged due to concerns about an increased risk of congestive heart failure. ACE inhibitors are helpful in CHF, give renal protective effect in diabetics with proteinuria, and are likely protective post-MI. Evidence is accumulating that angiotensin II receptor blockers provide these same benefits. Beta blockers are indicated post-MI, often in CHF, and in various tachyarrhythmia settings; they may help prevent migraines and treat essential tremor (which typically involves both hands from the outset in contrast to the tremor of Parkinson's disease).

438–440. The answers are 438-d, 439-b, 440-a. (*JNC 7 Express, pp 18–19. Kasper, pp 1472–1480.*) Diuretics predispose to hyperuricemia and therefore acute gout, the condition described in the first of these three questions; they can exacerbate hyperglycemia and must be used carefully in diabetics. Noncardioselective beta blockers are contraindicated in asthma/COPD and may adversely affect peripheral vascular disease, which the patient in the second of these three scenarios is describing with his symptom of claudication; other cautions include acute or unstable CHF, bradyarrhythmias, and diabetes (due to inhibition of usual sympathetic responses to hypoglycemia). ACE inhibitors and angiotensin II receptor blockers are contraindicated in the second and third trimesters of pregnancy, the underlying situation in the third of these three questions, due to the potential for fetal anomalies and death.

441–444. The answers are 441-c, 442-e, 443-d, 444-c. (*Kasper, pp 959–961, 964–965.*) Recommendations for isoniazid treatment of latent tuberculosis infection to prevent active disease (formerly called *chemoprophylaxis*) include the following (based on tuberculin reaction, measured by induration, not erythema):

HIV-infected persons or others receiving immunosuppressive therapy, 5 mm or greater
Close contacts of tuberculosis patients, 5 mm or greater
Persons with fibrotic lesions on CXR, 5 mm or greater
Recently infected persons (2 years or less), 10 mm or greater
Persons with high-risk medical conditions, 10 mm or greater [includes diabetes mellitus, some hematologic and reticuloendothelial diseases, injectable drug use (HIV-negative), end-stage renal disease, rapid weight loss]
Low-risk group, 15 mm or greater

By these criteria, the HIV-infected person and the 60-year-old recent converter are both candidates for isoniazid treatment, with the duration of therapy typically being 9 months. The risk of developing active TB in the

HIV-infected group is up to 15% per year and in other recent converters about 3% within the year. INH treatment is most likely to be effective when infection (conversion) is recent. Consideration may be given to providing treatment to all those under age 35 with positive PPDs, since the incidence of INH hepatitis in this group is low. The 40-year-old male with a positive PPD does not fall into any category of INH treatment. In contrast, the new nursing home patient should get a second PPD placed in 2 weeks. About 15% of these patients will have a false-negative PPD on the first test, but a true-positive on the second. The treatment of choice for active pulmonary tuberculosis is usually a 2-month initial phase of four drugs (isoniazid, rifampin, pyrazinamide, and ethambutol) followed by a 4-month continuation phase of isoniazide plus rifampin.

Allergy and Immunology

Questions

DIRECTIONS: Each item below contains a question followed by suggested responses. Select the **one best** response to each question.

445. A 20-year-old female develops urticaria that lasts for 6 weeks and then resolves spontaneously. She gives no history of weight loss, fever, rash, or tremulousness. Physical exam shows no abnormalities. Which of the following is the most likely cause of the urticaria?

a. Connective tissue disease
b. Hyperthyroidism
c. Chronic infection
d. Not likely to be determined

446. A 20-year-old male is found to have weight loss and generalized lymphadenopathy. He has hypogammaglobulinemia with a normal distribution of immunoglobulin isotypes. Histologic exam of lymphoid tissue shows germinal center hyperplasia. A diagnosis of common variable immunodeficiency is made. Which of the following is correct?

a. The patient likely had symptoms in childhood
b. At least one parent is also afflicted with the disease
c. The patient may develop recurrent bronchitis and chronic idiopathic diarrhea
d. The patient should receive the standard vaccine protocol

447. A 25-year-old female complains of watery rhinorrhea and pruritus of the eyes and nose that occurs around the same season each year. Symptoms are not exacerbated by weather changes, emotion, or irritants. She is on no medications and is not pregnant. Which of the following statements is correct?

a. In this patient, symptoms are being produced by an IgE antibody against a specific allergen
b. The patient has vasomotor rhinitis
c. The patient's nasal turbinates are likely to be very red
d. Avoidance measures alone are almost always effective

448. A 20-year-old nursing student complains of asthma while on her surgical rotation. She has developed dermatitis of her hands. Symptoms are worsened when she is in the operating room. Which of the following is correct?

a. This is an allergic reaction that is always benign
b. The patient should be evaluated for latex allergy by skin testing
c. This syndrome is less common now than 10 years ago
d. Oral corticosteroid is indicated

449. A 30-year-old male develops skin rash, pruritus, and mild wheezing about 20 min after an intravenous pyelogram performed for the evaluation of renal stone symptoms. Which of the following is the best approach to diagnosis of this patient?

a. Perform 24-h urinary histamine measurement
b. Measure immunoglobulin E to radiocontrast media
c. Diagnose radiocontrast media sensitivity by history
d. Recommend intradermal skin testing

450. A 16-year-old woman develops wheezing and shortness of breath minutes after receiving ceftriaxone for gonorrhea. Which of the following is the treatment of choice for this patient?

a. Subcutaneous epinephrine for bronchospasm
b. Intravenous fluids
c. Prophylactic atropine
d. Diazepam to prevent seizures
e. Antihistamine

451. A 40-year-old white woman with a history of chronic otitis and sinusitis is found to have a serum IgA level of 1 mg/dL. All other immunoglobulin classes are found to be normal. Which of the following statements is correct?

a. She may suffer an anaphylactic reaction following the administration of serum products
b. Clinical improvement follows regular infusions of fresh plasma
c. Infection with *Giardia* should suggest a different diagnosis
d. The disease is more common in blacks and Asians than it is in whites
e. An associated autoimmune disorder would be very rare

452. A 55-year-old farmer develops recurrent cough, dyspnea, fever, and myalgia several hours after entering his barn. Which of the following statements is true?

a. Testing of pulmonary function several hours after an exposure will most likely reveal an obstructive pattern
b. Immediate-type IgE hypersensitivity is involved in the pathogenesis of his illness
c. The etiological agents may well be thermophilic actinomycete antigens
d. Demonstrating precipitable antibodies to the offending antigen confirms the diagnosis of hypersensitivity pneumonitis

453. A 35-year-old woman is concerned that she may be allergic to some foods. She believes that she gets a rash several hours after eating small amounts of peanuts. In evaluating this concern, which of the following is correct?

a. At least 30% of the adult population is allergic to some food substance
b. Symptoms occur hours after ingestion of the food substance
c. The foods most likely to cause allergic reactions include egg, milk, seafood, nuts, and soybeans
d. The organ systems most frequently involved in allergic reactions to foods in adults are the respiratory and cardiovascular systems
e. Immunotherapy is a proven therapy for food allergies

454. A 32-year-old woman experiences a severe anaphylactic reaction following a sting from a hornet. Which of the following statements is correct?

a. She would not have a similar reaction to a sting from a yellow jacket
b. She would have a prior history of an adverse reaction to an insect sting
c. Adults are unlikely to die as a result of an insect sting compared to children with the same history
d. She should be skin-tested with venom antigens and, if positive, immunotherapy should be started

DIRECTIONS: Each group of questions below consists of lettered options followed by a set of numbered items. For each numbered item, select the **one** lettered option with which it is **most** closely associated. Each lettered option may be used once, more than once, or not at all.

Questions 455–457

For each clinical description, select the one most likely immunologic deficiency.

a. Wiskott-Aldrich syndrome
b. Ataxia telangiectasia
c. DiGeorge syndrome
d. Immunoglobulin A deficiency
e. Severe combined immunodeficiency
f. C1 inhibitor deficiency
g. Decay-accelerating factor deficiency

455. A 16-year-old male has recurrent episodes of nonpruritic, nonerythematous angioedema. There is a family history of angioedema. The patient has also complained of recurring abdominal pain.

456. A 30-year-old male of European descent has episodes of anemia secondary to hemolysis. He has also been diagnosed with venous thrombosis. On evaluation of anemia there is hemoglobinuria and elevated LDH.

457. An 18-year-old male gives history that inludes episodes of eczema and recurrent sinus and gastrointestinal infections. His platelet count is 90,000/μL.

Questions 458–460

For each patient, select the most likely immunologic deficiency.

a. Complement deficiency C5–C9
b. Selective IgA deficiency
c. Post-splenectomy
d. Neutropenia
e. Interleukin 12 receptor deficit
f. Microbicidal leukocyte defect
g. Phagocyte immune deficit
h. Congenital T-cell deficit

458. A 30-year-old male has developed fever, chills, and neck stiffness. Cerebrospinal fluid shows gram-negative diplococci. He has had a past episode of sepsis with meningococemia. _C_

459. A 22-year-old male has been healthy except for abdominal surgery after an auto accident. He is admitted with clinical signs of pneumonia and meningitis. Cultures of blood, sputum, and cerebrospinal fluid grow gram-positive diplococci. _C_

460. A 40-year-old with chronic myelogenous leukemia has had several episodes of sepsis after chemotherapy. _D_

Allergy and Immunology

Answers

445. The answer is d. *(Kasper, pp 1951–1952.)* Urticaria, also known as hives, presents as well-circumscribed wheals with raised serpiginous borders. The process may be triggered by a specific antigen such as food, drugs, or pollen. It may also be bradykinin-mediated, such as in hereditary angioedema, or complement-mediated, as in necrotizing vasculitis. However, in the great majority of patients with urticaria, a cause is never found. Some do have underlying illnesses such as chronic infection, myeloproliferative disease, collagen vascular disease, or hyperthyroidism. There is no evidence for underlying disease in this patient.

446. The answer is c. *(Kasper, p 1944.)* Patients with common variable immunodeficiency syndrome usually develop recurrent or chronic infections of the respiratory or gastrointestinal tract. Patients have hypogammaglobulinemia, often with associated T cell abnormalities. Diarrhea can be idiopathic, with malabsorption, or secondary to chronic infection such as giardiasis. There is no typical genetic predisposition, although clusters in families do occur. Symptoms generally do not occur until the second or third decade of life, but also may first present in the older patient. Patients with common variable immunodeficiency syndrome should not receive live vaccines such as those for mumps, rubella, or polio.

447. The answer is a. *(Kasper, pp 1954–1955.)* Allergic rhinitis is caused by allergens that trigger a local hypersensitivity reaction. Specific IgE antibodies are produced and attach to circulating mast cells or basophils. Mast cell degranulation leads to a cascade of inflammatory mediators. Vasomotor rhinitis, the second most common cause of rhinitis after allergic disease, is usually perennial and is not associated with itching. In allergic rhinitis, nasal turbinates appear pale and boggy. Avoidance measures alone are often ineffective. Antihistamines and intranasal corticosteroids are usually recommended.

448. The answer is b. *(Kasper, pp 289–290.)* Latex allergy has become an increasingly recognized problem. This is an IgE-mediated sensitivity to latex products, particularly surgical gloves. Patients present with localized urticaria at the site of contact, but can also have generalized urticaria, flushing, wheezing, laryngeal edema, and hypotension. A scratch test with latex extract is the most sensitive approach to diagnosis. The test must be done with caution since anaphylaxis can occur. Education and avoidance of latex products is the best approach to management.

449. The answer is c. *(Cochran, pp 28–31.)* Signs and symptoms of radiocontrast media sensitivity include tachycardia, wheezing, urticaria, facial edema, bradycardia, and hypotension. When these occur within 20 min of the injection of a radiocontrast agent, the diagnosis is made by history. No routine laboratory abnormalities are diagnostic or predictive. Specific immunoglobulin E antibodies have not been identified, and no specific skin test is available.

450. The answer is a. *(Kasper, p 1950.)* Subcutaneous epinephrine is recommended for bronchospasm and anaphylaxis. (For severe bronchospasm, intravenous epinephrine might be used in this patient, who does not have contraindications.) Intravenous fluids would be recommended only when hypotension is present. Atropine is given only in the setting of bradycardia. Diazepam is used when seizures occur acutely as part of the hypersensitivity reaction. Antihistamines are not helpful for the naphyactic reaction.

451. The answer is a. *(Kasper, p 1944.)* IgA deficiency occurs in approximately 1 in 700 births. It is much more common in whites than in blacks or Asians. (The incidence in Japan is 1 in 18,500.) IgA-deficient patients produce autoantibodies. Some develop high levels of antibody to IgA, which can result in anaphylactic reaction when transfused with normal blood or blood products. Failure to produce IgA antibody results in recurrent upper respiratory tract infections in more than 50% of affected patients. Chronic diarrhea and *Giardia* infection are common problems. IgA-deficient patients frequently have autoimmune disorders, atopic problems, and malabsorption and eventually develop pulmonary disease. IgA cannot be effectively replaced with exogenous immunoglobulin.

452. The answer is c. *(Kasper, pp 1516–1517.)* Hypersensitivity pneumonitis is characterized by an immunologic inflammatory reaction in response to inhaling organic dusts, the most common of which are thermophilic actinomycetes, fungi, and avian proteins. In the acute form of the illness, exposure to the offending antigen is intense. Cough, dyspnea, fever, chills, and myalgia, which typically occur 4 to 8 hours after exposure, are the presenting symptoms. In the subacute form, antigen exposure is moderate, chills and fever are usually absent, and cough, anorexia, weight loss, and dyspnea dominate the presentation. In the chronic form of hypersensitivity pneumonitis, progressive dyspnea, weight loss, and anorexia are seen; pulmonary fibrosis is a noted complication. The finding of IgG antibody to the offending antigen is universal, although it may be present in asymptomatic patients as well and is therefore not diagnostic. While peripheral T cell, B cell, and monocyte counts are normal, a suppressor cell functional defect can be demonstrated in these patients. Inhalation challenge with the suspected antigen and concomitant testing of pulmonary function help to confirm the diagnosis. Therapy involves avoidance; steroids are administered in severe cases. Bronchodilators and antihistamines are not effective.

453. The answer is c. *(Novartis Foundation, pp 161–171.)* Food allergy is an IgE-mediated reaction to antigens in food. It is caused by glycoproteins found in shellfish, peanuts, eggs, milk, nuts, and soybeans. Symptoms occur within minutes of ingestion in most patients. The incidence of true food allergy in the general population is uncertain but is likely to be about 1% of patients—less than might be generally perceived. Studies have demonstrated that exclusive breastfeeding can decrease the incidence of allergies to food in infants genetically predisposed to developing them. Food allergens cause symptoms most commonly expressed in the gastrointestinal tract and the skin. In addition, respiratory and (in severe reactions) cardiovascular symptoms may occur. Food allergic reactions are diagnosed by the medical history, skin tests, or radioallergosorbent tests (RASTs), and elimination diets. The best test, however, remains the double-blind, placebo-controlled food challenge. If the diagnosis of a food allergy is confirmed, the only proven therapy is avoidance of the offending food. At present, there is no role for immunotherapy in the treatment of food allergy.

454. The answer is d. (*Kasper, pp 2605–2606.*) The incidence of insect sting allergy is difficult to determine. Approximately 40 deaths per year occur as a result of *Hymenoptera* stings. Additional fatalities undoubtedly occur and are unknowingly attributed to other causes. Both atopic and nonatopic persons experience reactions to insect stings. The responses range from large local reactions with erythema and swelling at the sting site to acute anaphylaxis. The majority of fatal reactions occur in adults, with most persons having had no previous reaction to a stinging insect. Reactions can occur with the first sting and usually begin within 15 min. Enzymes, biogenic amines, and peptides are the allergens present in the insects' venom that provoke allergic reactions. Venoms are commercially available for testing and treatment. Within the *Vespidae* family, which consists of hornets, yellow jackets, and wasps, cross-sensitivity to the various insect venoms occurs. The honeybee, which belongs to the *Apis* family, does not show cross-reactivity with the vespids. Venom immunotherapy is indicated for patients with a history of sting anaphylaxis and positive skin tests.

455–457. The answers are 455-f, 456-g, 457-a. (*Kasper, pp 616, 1946, 1952.*) C1 inhibitor deficiency prevents the proper regulation of activated C1. As a consequence, levels of C2 and C4—substrates of C1—are also low. Recurrent angioedema is the result of uncontrolled action of other serum proteins normally controlled by C1 inhibitor. The disease may be acquired but is also autosomal dominant due to a deficiency of C1 inhibitor. There is no pruritus or urticarial lesions. Recurrent gastrointestinal attacks of colic commonly occur.

Decay-accelerating factor is a membrane-anchored protein that inhibits complement activation of host tissue. Deficiency predisposes to erythrocyte lysis that results in paroxysmal nocturnal hemoglobinuria. PNH should be suspected in patients with unexplained hemolytic anemia and evidence of intravascular hemolysis (such as hemoglobinuria, hemoglobinemeia, and elevated LDH). Venous thrombosis is a common complication in those of European descent.

Wiskott-Aldrich syndrome is an X-linked recessive disorder associated with thrombocytopenia, eczema, and recurrent infection. There is an increased incidence of lymphoreticular neoplasm. The disease is the result of an abnormal protein caused by a mutation in the WASP gene. It may

463. An 82-year-old man complains of 2 h of severe chest pain that occurred while he was playing tennis. Blood pressure on admission is 140/70, and heart rate is 110. There are no signs of congestive heart failure. Pulses are all palpable, and abdominal exam is normal. Neurologic exam is normal, and stool is guaiac-negative. There is no history of gastrointestinal bleeding, previous stroke, head trauma, or major surgery. There is no history of vascular disease or liver disease. ECG shows ST segment elevation of 3 mm in leads V_1 through V_3, with three premature ventricular beats per minute. Which of the following is the initial treatment of choice?

a. Prophylactic lidocaine
b. Thrombolytic therapy and aspirin
c. Heparin
d. Aspirin alone

464. A 65-year-old man has had symptoms of progressive cognitive dysfunction over a 1-year period. Memory and calculation ability are worsening. The patient has also had episodes of paranoia and delusions. Antipsychotic medication resulted in extrapyramidal signs and was stopped. The patient has recently complained of several months of visual hallucinations. There is no history of alcohol abuse. Which of the following is the most likely diagnosis?

a. Lewy body dementia
b. Alzheimer's disease
c. Early parkinsonism
d. Delirium

465. An 80-year-old nursing home patient has become increasingly confused and unstable on her feet. On one occasion she has wandered outside the nursing home. In considering the issue of restraints for this individual, which of the following is correct?

a. A geri-chair would provide the best approach to safety and restraint
b. Physical restraints are the best method to prevent falls
c. Restraints cause many complications and increase the risk of falls
d. Sedative medication should be used instead of restraints

466. A 75-year-old woman who is living independently seeks advice about exercise programs. She has mild hypertension but is otherwise in good health with no other risk factors for cardiovascular disease. Which of the following statements is supported by current data?

a. Walking can reduce mortality from cardiovascular disease and help prevent falls
b. Tai chi has become popular in the elderly but results in falls
c. This patient would require stress testing before beginning a walking program
d. Only high-intensity exercise has been shown to have long-standing benefits

467. A frail 80-year-old nursing home resident has had several episodes of syncope, all of which have occurred while she was returning to her room after breakfast. She complains of light-headedness and states she feels cold and weak. She takes nitroglycerin in the morning for a history of chest pain, but denies recent chest pain or shortness of breath. Which of the following is the most likely method of diagnosis?

a. Cardiac catheterization
b. Postprandial blood pressure monitoring
c. Holter monitoring
d. CT scan

468. A 90-year-old male has a history of myocardial infarction, early congestive heart failure, and episodes of atrial fibrillation. Which of the following medications should be avoided for the indication given?

a. A beta blocker after myocardial infarction
b. Angiotensin-converting enzyme inhibitor in left ventricular systolic dysfunction
c. Warfarin in chronic atrial fibrillation
d. Digoxin in early signs of congestive heart failure

469. A 78-year-old male complains of slowly progressive hearing loss. He finds it particularly difficult to hear his grandchildren and to appreciate conversation in a crowded restaurant. On exam, ear canal and tympanic membranes are normal. Audiology testing finds bilateral upper-frequency hearing loss with difficulties in speech discrimination. Which of the following is the most likely diagnosis?

a. Presbycusis
b. Cerumen impaction
c. Ménière's disease
d. Chronic otitis media

470. A 90-year-old male complains of nonspecific weakness, some shortness of breath on exertion, and poor sleep. In evaluating this patient, which of the following physiologic parameters does not change with age?

a. Creatinine clearance
b. Forced expiratory volume
c. Hematocrit
d. Heart rate response to stress
e. Hours of REM sleep

471. A 65-year-old male who has not had routine medical care presents for a physical exam and is found to have a blood pressure of 165/80. He has no other risk factors for heart disease. He is not obese and walks 1 mile a day. Physical exam shows no retinopathy, normal cardiac exam including point of maximal impulse, and normal pulses. There is no abdominal bruit, and neurological exam is normal. ECG, electrolytes, blood sugar, and urinalysis are also normal. Repeat visit 2 weeks later shows blood pressure to be unchanged. Which of the following is the best next step in management?

a. Do a workup for secondary causes, including intravenous pyelogram
b. Begin therapy with a low-dose diuretic
c. Follow patient; avoid toxicity of antihypertensive agents
d. Begin therapy with a beta blocker

472. A 65-year-old male inquires about the pneumonia vaccine. He has a friend who died of pneumonia. The patient is in good health without underlying disease. Which of the following is the most appropriate management of this patient?

a. Recommend the pneumococcal vaccine and check on the status of other immunizations, particularly tetanus vaccination
b. Inform the patient that he has no risk factors for pneumonia
c. Report that the present pneumonia vaccine does not work
d. Emphasize that the influenza vaccine is more important

473. This 80-year-old white male is being evaluated as part of an annual physical exam. On examination there is a large plaque on the left shoulder that is well demarcated, hyperkeratotic, and oily to palpation. It appears to be "stuck on." It's surface includes keratin plugs. Which of the following is the most appropriate next step?

a. Biopsy to rule out melanoma
b. Advice about sun exposure and actinic keratosis
c. Reassurance of the benign nature of this seborrheic keratosis
d. Removal of basal cell carcinoma

474. A 67-year-old male asks for advice about vaccination with the influenza vaccine on a routine visit in the fall. He is ambulatory, in good health, and does not have cardiac or pulmonary disease. There is some shortage of the influenza inactivated vaccine for the year. Which of the following is the best approach to this vaccination?

a. Give the intranasal live vaccine if it is more available than the inactivated vaccine
b. Assure the patient that vaccination against influenza is not mandatory since there is no underlying disease
c. Vaccinate the patient with the inactivated vaccine unless he is allergic to eggs
d. Treat the patient with amantadine at the first sign of an influenza outbreak

DIRECTIONS: Each group of questions below consists of lettered options followed by a set of numbered items. For each numbered item, select the **one** lettered option with which it is **most** closely associated. Each lettered option may be used once, more than once, or not at all.

Questions 475–477
   Match the patient with the most likely type of urinary incontinence
a. Stress incontinence
b. Urge incontinence
c. Overflow incontinence
d. Functional incontinence
e. Mixed incontinence
f. Normal physiologic functioning of old age

475. A 70-year-old woman complains of having problems with leaking of urine in small amounts. This occurs when laughing or coughing. It has also occurred while bending or exercising. The patient has five children who are concerned about her urinary problems.

476. An 80-year-old male has been admitted to a nursing home after a stroke. He has a hemiparesis and expressive aphasia. After 2 weeks he is still unable to make it to the bathroom. Urodynamic testing shows no abnormalities.

477. This 85-year-old male has a history of long-standing diabetes mellitus and prostatic hypertrophy. He complains of dribbling urine. There is a sense of incomplete voiding and of a decrease in urinary stream. Postvoiding residual is 300 mL.

Geriatrics

Answers

461. The answer is d. *(Kasper, pp 48, 2400.)* The best course would be to continue the donepezil and see if it slows progression of cognitive function loss based on mini–mental status exam or family assessment. The success of the intervention needs to be evaluated over a longer time period, realizing that success may mean maintaining baseline function. The anticholinesterase inhibitors do not prevent plaque formation. Increasing the dose is rarely helpful and often causes side effects. There is no data to suggest that one anticholinesterase inhibitor works better than another.

462. The answer is c. *(Kane, pp 267–268.)* In addition to physical therapy, the best symptomatic treatment would be acetaminophen because it is frequently effective in providing pain relief and has an excellent safety profile in the elderly. Nonsteroidals should be avoided, at least initially, because they tend to cause gastrointestinal upset and impairment of renal function. Intraarticular steroids are indicated for large effusions in joints unresponsive to first-line therapy. Arthroplasty is highly effective in treating osteoarthritis of a single joint and is not contraindicated in the elderly. Such surgery is usually considered after attempts at physical therapy, education, and pain relief with pharmacotherapy.

463. The answer is b. *(Kane, p 295.)* The patient has clinical and ECG evidence for acute myocardial infarction. He has no contraindications to thrombolytic therapy. (Age per se is not a contraindication to thrombolytic therapy.) Thirty-day mortality is markedly decreased for elderly patients with acute MI treated with aspirin and thrombolytic therapy. Many elderly patients, of course, will have contraindications to thrombolytics, particularly gastrointestinal bleeding, recent stroke, head injury, or surgery. Aspirin alone is not as effective in reducing mortality. Antiarrthymic agents do not reduce mortality and have pronounced side effects in the elderly. Heparin should be given following thrombolytic therapy.

464. The answer is a. *(Kasper, pp 52, 2402–2403.)* Lewy body dementia has been recently recognized as a specific type of dementia different from

Alzheimer's disease or Parkinson's disease. On autopsy there is evidence of Lewy bodies throughout the brain, including the cortex. Mild parkinsonism may or may not be present. Paranoia and delusions are more common than in Alzheimer's disease, and treatment with antipsychotic drugs characteristically worsens the underlying condition. The visual hallucinations are the most characteristic clinical symptom, making the diagnosis of Alzheimer's disease less likely. Delirium is an acute confusional state that would not present with progressive cognitive deterioration or repeated hallucinations over time.

465. The answer is c. (*Kane, p 438.*) Restraints are being used less and less in nursing homes as their complications and alternatives become more appreciated. The four D's—**d**econditioning, **d**epression, **d**isorientation, and **d**ecubiti—are all complications of restraints. A geri-chair is just another form of physical restraint, which promotes the same difficulties. Effective alternatives to restraints usually require an individual care plan. In this case, alarm bells for the institution's exits and evaluation of the patient's gait would be important. Sedation leads to complications such as pneumonia and may, in fact, also promote falls.

466. The answer is a. (*Kasper, p 53.*) Walking is the most common exercise in the elderly and has been shown to reduce mortality from coronary artery disease and decrease the incidence of falls. In one study, a rigorous walking program of 2 miles a day reduced coronary artery disease events by 50%. Tai chi exercises, which consist of a sequence of movements used in martial arts, have actually been shown to reduce the incidence of falls in older patients. Exercise need not be high-intensity to have benefits; moderate-intensity activity for 30 min produces most of the health benefits of daily exercise. Judgment dictates the degree of medical screening and the use of exercise stress testing in elderly patients who are beginning an exercise program. A walking program does not require such screening. Exercise stress testing has been recommended by some experts for elderly patients with two or more risk factors for heart disease.

467. The answer is b. (*Kasper, p 50.*) Postprandial hypotension has been increasingly recognized in the frail elderly. Postprandial reduction in systolic blood pressure in the elderly is common. In one study, a quarter of all patients had a reduction in systolic blood pressure of greater than 20 mmHg. Much of the decrease is due to splanchnic blood pooling. Those on nitrates and other drugs that cause postural hypotension are at greatest risk. Older patients with this condition should avoid large meals. Diagnosis is confirmed by monitoring blood pressure after eating. Cardiac ischemia or arrythmia cannot be ruled out but are less likely to cause the symptoms described. Arrhythmia is more likely to be of sudden onset but could be evaluated by continuous monitoring later in the workup. CT scan is rarely helpful in the evaluation of syncope in a patient without focal neurologic findings.

468. The answer is d. *(Kane, pp 281–300.)* All medications should be carefully considered in the elderly with respect to side effects and drug interactions. However, some medications are in fact used too infrequently in the elderly because of side effect concerns. Beta blockers prolong survival in the elderly after myocardial infarction, and have probably been used too infrequently in the elderly after MI. Similarly, ACE inhibitors have a beneficial effect on mortality and functional status in the elderly with systolic dysfunction. They should be prescribed unless there are contraindications such as intolerance, renal insufficiency, elevated serum potassium, or hypotension. Warfarin reduces the risk of thromboembolic events in the elderly with atrial fibrillation. It is estimated that warfarin could prevent an additional 40,000 strokes per year in patients with atrial fibrillation, most of whom are elderly. Digoxin is rarely a drug of choice for heart failure in the elderly patient. In general, it is a drug to avoid in the elderly because of its toxic-to-therapeutic ratio and tendency for drug interactions.

469. The answer is a. *(Kane, pp 345–351.)* Presbycusis is the most common cause of sensorineural hearing loss in the elderly. Probably the result of cochlear damage over time, it is characterized by bilateral high-frequency hearing loss above 2000 Hz. Diminished speech discrimination is more apparent compared to other causes of hearing loss. Both Ménière's disease and chronic otitis media are common causes of hearing loss in the elderly; they usually present as unilateral hearing loss. Otoscopy should always be used to rule out hearing loss due to cerumen impaction in the elderly patient.

470. The answer is c. *(Kasper, pp 43–49.)* Hematocrit does not vary with age, and elderly patients with anemia require workup to define the disease process. Lung elasticity decreases with age, resulting in some change over time in pulmonary function test. Creatinine clearance decreases with age, as do heart rate response to stress and number of hours of REM sleep.

471. The answer is b. *(Kane, pp 284–289.)* There is now general agreement that systolic hypertension in the elderly should be treated and that low-dose thiazide diuretic is the initial regimen of choice in the elderly. Treatment reduces the risk of stroke and cardiovascular events, and side effects appear to be minimal. Atenolol is generally recommended as second-step therapy. Workup for secondary causes is not indicated, as they are less common in the elderly; however, such a workup may be appropriate if hypertension is refractory to medication. Weight loss and exercise might be initiated prior to antihypertensive medication in a patient with mild systolic hypertension who is obese or sedentary.

472. The answer is a. *(Kasper, pp 813–814.)* The pneumococcal vaccine is currently recommended for all patients over the age of 65 because age per se is a risk factor for mortality due to pneumococcal infection. The vaccine is safe, and the vaccination program for the elderly is cost-effective. The importance of the annual influenza vaccine should also be explained to the patient. If the visit is during influenza season, both vaccines should be given at the same time. Tetanus vaccination booster is also recommended in the elderly patient who has not had a booster vaccine in 10 years.

473. The answer is c. *(Kasper, pp 285, 502.)* The lesion described is characteristic of seborrheic keratosis, which is an extremely common lesion in older patients. The waxy, stuck-on-appearing lesion with keratin plugs is so identifiable that it requires no further workup. It is a benign growth of normal epithelial cells. Melanomas are usually asymmetric with irregular borders and color variegation. Basal cell carcinoma usually presents as a pearly translucent nodule with telangiectasia. Actinic keratoses, a precursor to squamous cell carcinoma, have a reddish, scaly appearance and are usually erythematous papules.

474. The answer is c. *(Kane, pp 97, 98, 101.)* All patients over the age of 65 are high priority to receive the influenza vaccine whether they have underlying disease or not. Most deaths from influenza occur in the over-65 age group. Currently, the live attenuated intranasal vaccine is not approved in the elderly patient population. Amantadine can be started in a patient who has not been vaccinated and is in the midst of an epidemic. However, especially in the elderly, efforts to vaccinate should occur in October or November, prior to influenza activity.

475–477. The answers are 475-a, 476-d, 477-c. *(Kane, pp 188–195, 500–507.)* The 70-year-old woman with episodes of leaking small amounts of urine while laughing or coughing has stress incontinence. Stress incontinence occurs when the internal urethral sphincter fails to remain closed in response to increasing intraabdominal pressure caused by laughing, coughing, or lifting. The problem is usually seen in postmenopausal women who have weakening of their pubococcygeus muscle after multiple childbirths.

The 80-year-old male with a stroke history is most likely to have functional incontinence. This often occurs after a major illness or after transfer to a nursing home. The patient cannot notify caregivers about urge to urinate. The patient just cannot make it to the bathroom because of debility, confusion, poor vision, or poor hearing. Sometimes sedative medications contribute to the problem.

Diabetes and prostatic hypertrophy may be contributing to this 85-year-old man's overflow incontinence. Overflow incontinence occurs when there is a mechanical or functional obstruction at the bladder outlet. This leads to overfill of the bladder and leakage with detrusor contraction. A similar picture can occur in a diabetic with an atonic bladder.

Women's Health

Questions

DIRECTIONS: Each item below contains a question followed by suggested responses. Select the **one best** response to each question.

478. A 20-year-old sexually active female presents for an annual exam. She tells you she has had four sexual partners in the past, she has participated in unprotected intercourse sometimes, and her age at first coitus was 15. She has a 5-pack-year tobacco history. Her family history is positive for early coronary artery disease in her father and paternal grandfather. On physical exam, she is overweight. Otherwise her exam is normal. On pelvic exam, there are no cervical lesions, and a Pap smear is obtained. Several days later, the Pap smear result is reported as a low-grade squamous intraepithelial lesion (LGSIL). Which of the following infectious agents is most likely associated with this result?

a. Human papillomavirus (HPV)
b. Herpes simplex virus
c. Chlamydia
d. Trichomonas vaginalis
e. Group B streptococcus

479. An 18-year-old G1P1 presents to your office with the results of an abnormal Pap smear dated 1 month ago. She tells you that she had one Pap smear prior to this one and it was normal. She reports having had four sexual partners since beginning sexual activity at age 15. Upon reviewing the Pap smear result you find it is reported as low-grade squamous intraepithelial lesion (LGSIL). Based upon this information, which of the following is the most appropriate next step in the management of this abnormal pap smear?

a. Have further evaluation of cervical abnormality
b. Repeat pap at next annual Pap smear
c. Have a repeat Pap smear if and when she changes sexual partners
d. Have Pap smear repeated every 3 years
e. No further evaluation is needed

480. A 60-year-old white female presents for an office visit. Her mother recently broke her hip, and the patient is concerned about her own risk for osteoporosis. She weighs 165 lb and is 5 ft 6 in. tall. She has a 50-pack-year history of tobacco use. Medications include a multivitamin and levothyroxine 50 µg/d. Her exercise regimen includes mowing the lawn and taking care of the garden. She took hormone replacement therapy for 6 years after menopause, which occurred at age 49. Which of the following tests related to osteoporosis, if any, is appropriate for this patient?

a. Nuclear medicine bone scan
b. Dual x-ray absorptiometry (Dexa scan)
c. No testing is required at this time
d. Peripheral bone densitometry

481. A 55-year-old Asian female presents for her annual exam. She is a nonsmoker and otherwise healthy. Her medications include a multivitamin per day. She reports walking 2 miles per day at least 5 days per week. She is 5 ft 2 in. and 110 lb. In addition to recommending a test to screen for osteoporosis you also recommend which of the following to help maintain bone health?

a. Fluoride supplementation
b. Calcium supplementation
c. Changing her current exercise routine
d. Restarting hormone replacement therapy
e. Vitamin E supplementation

482. You are volunteering at a health fair, working in the osteoporosis screening booth. A 62-year-old white female stops by to ask if she needs to be evaluated for osteoporosis. In addition to being a white female and postmenopausal, which of the following factors would increase her risk of osteoporosis?

a. Excessive supplementation of vitamin C
b. Hypothyroidism
c. Obesity
d. Use of hormone replacement therapy
e. Family history of osteoporosis

483. A 50-year-old woman presents with a vague complaint of fatigue and dyspnea on exertion. The dyspnea occurs with activities such as vacuuming or climbing the stairs in her home. Resting for 10 to 15 min relieves the symptoms. The patient noticed this about 1 to 2 months ago. She denies chest pain, orthopnea, paroxysmal nocturnal dyspnea, or recent respiratory infection. Past medical history is significant for hypertension for 10 years and hyperlipidemia for 5 years. Her medications include hydrochlorothiazide. She tries to watch her cholesterol intake. Social history is negative for tobacco use. She does recall a family history of heart attacks and strokes in her mother's family, but cannot give details. On physical exam, lungs are clear bilaterally and cardiovascular exam is unremarkable without murmurs. A left carotid bruit is noted. ECG reveals poor R wave progression in V_1 through V_2 and nonspecific ST-T wave changes anterolaterally. Chest x-ray is normal. Pulse oximetry is 97%. Laboratory evaluation shows a normal complete blood count, cholesterol 250, HDL 29 mg/dL, LDL 160 mg/dL, glucose (random) 250/dL. Which of the following disease processes is most likely contributing to this patient's symptoms?

a. Coronary artery disease
b. Pneumonia
c. Medication side effects
d. Anxiety disorder

484. A 52-year-old black female presents to your office with complaints of an occasional uncomfortable feeling in her chest. She has noticed the chest pain occurring over the past 6 months. The pain usually starts when she gets angry or is hurrying from the parking lot into the office building where she works. The pain is sharp and located in the center of her chest. Sometimes it is associated with shortness of breath. It lasts less than 1 to 2 minutes. Upon reviewing her medical history you note she has poorly controlled hypertension and glucose intolerance. She tells you she does not perform any regular exercise and has gained 20 lb in the past 2 years. On exam, her blood pressure is 150/94, and BMI is 31. Medications include hydrochlorthiazide and lisinopril. Which of the following actions would be most helpful in diagnosing the cause of this patient's chest pain?

a. Discontinuation of current medication
b. Pulmonary function testing
c. Graded exercise treadmill stress test
d. Graded exercise treadmill stress test with thallium scanning
e. No further test necessary, reassure the patient

485. A 55-year-old white female presents for an annual exam. Medical history is significant for hypertension. She is a nonsmoker. Family history is negative for coronary artery disease. She has no acute complaints. She weighs 80 kg and is 1.65 m tall. BP is 150/100, cholesterol 250 mg/dL, triglycerides 300 mg/dL, HDL 30 mg/dL, and LDL 160 mg/dL. This patient's calculated body mass index (BMI) is which of the following?

a. 33
b. 29
c. 25
d. 22.4
e. 20

486. A 19-year-old female presents to your office with complaints of dizziness when she stands up. She denies any associated symptoms. Review of systems reveals no recent illness, weight loss, or weight gain. Her last menstrual cycle was 1 year ago. The patient states she is not using any medications or over-the-counter supplements. On physical exam, you note a very thin white female, weight 102 lb, height 5 ft 7 in., PR 45. Skin exam reveals no ecchymosis, but lanugo hair is noted. BP lying down is 100/60, standing is 80/50; PR lying down is 45, standing is 70. The patient reports a slight dizzy feeling when standing up. You suspect this patient has an eating disorder. In addition to an EKG and laboratory evaluation, you document a goal BMI for this patient as which of the following?

a. 17.5 to 23
b. 26.0 to 31.0
c. 15 to 20
d. 24.5 to 30
e. 18.5 to 24.9

487. A 28-year-old female complains of fatigue and a sense of fullness at the base of her neck. She has no significant past medical history, gave birth to a healthy infant 4 months ago, and is only taking oral contraceptives. On exam, vital signs are pulse 88, blood pressure 110/66, temperature 98.6°F, and respirations 12. You note a homogeneously enlarged thyroid gland and a very mild fine tremor. The rest of the exam is within normal limits. Laboratory evaluation reveals the following:

WBC: 7.8
Hgb: 12.3
Hct: 36
Plt: 220
Na: 138
K: 4.0
Cl: 106
CO_2: 26
BUN: 12
Creatinine: 0.7
TSH: 0.01
T_4: 19
Antithyroid antibody test: elevated

Preliminary diagnosis is consistent with which of the following?

a. Thyrotoxicosis factitia
b. Subacute thyroiditis
c. Toxic multinodular goiter
d. Postpartum thyroiditis
e. Struma ovarii

488. A 51-year-old female presents to your office with questions about whether hormone replacement therapy (HRT) is "dangerous." She states she heard this on the news and read about it in a women's magazine. She denies ever having symptoms of menopause. She has hypertension, but is otherwise healthy. Her family history is negative for breast cancer and cardiovascular disease.

You explain to this patient that there was recently a large study about HRT, "The Women's Health Initiative Study," and according to this study you recommend which of the following for this patient?

a. Start HRT for cardiovascular protection
b. HRT is not indicated for this patient
c. Start vaginal estrogen cream
d. Start HRT for breast cancer risk reduction

489. A 25-year-old white female presents to your office for an annual exam. She is a G2P2 and had a bilateral tubal ligation after her last child was born (3 years ago). LMP: 2 weeks ago. On review of systems she describes two to three headaches per month for the past year, usually unilateral and occasionally associated with nausea. The headaches last for several hours. She denies visual changes or other neurological changes when the headaches occur. She tells you she used to have migraine headaches in high school, but they stopped when she was about 20. When you question her about triggers for her headache she states she has not noted foods, alcohol, stress, or fatigue contributing to onset. She does state her headaches usually happen within the same several-day period and are not spread out over the month. Her last bout with the headaches was about 2½ weeks ago. Which of the following is the most likely diagnosis?

a. Tension headache
b. Cluster headache
c. Sinus headache
d. Classic migraine
e. Menstrual migraine

490. A 21-year-old female presents with complaints of fatigue and difficulty swallowing. She describes the difficulty swallowing as a choking sensation that occurs randomly and not with eating. She denies elevated temperature, chills, or nausea and vomiting. She states she is having some difficulty sleeping at night. She is 28 weeks pregnant with her first child. You note she is wearing long sleeves in warm weather and she has bruising on her forearms and left lateral thoracic area. An appropriate way to explore your concerns with the patient would be to ask which of the following questions?

a. "Do you know how you got these bruises?"
b. "Who hit you?"
c. "How long has your partner been abusing you?"
d. "I will have to report these injuries to the appropriate authorities if you can't explain them."

491. A 24-week pregnant female presents with complaints of dysuria. A dipstick urinalysis in your office reveals 2+ leukocyte esterase, trace blood, no protein, no glucose, and 2+ nitrites. You send the urine to the laboratory for culture and sensitivity but want to start empiric treatment for the patient's symptoms. Which of the following medications is most appropriate?

a. Ciprofloxacin
b. Cephalexin
c. Trimethoprim-sulfamethoxazole
d. Tetracycline
e. Gentamicin

492. One month after an unremarkable vaginal delivery, a 34-year-old G1P1 is referred to you by her obstetrician due to the onset of fatigue, dyspnea, and lower extremity edema. By history, physical examination, and testing (including cardiac echocardiogram and chest x-ray), you make the diagnosis of peripartum cardiomyopathy. Which of the following is correct?

a. Peripartum cardiomyopathy may occur unexpectedly years after pregnancy and delivery
b. The postpartum state will require a different therapeutic approach than typical treatment for dilated cardiomyopathy
c. Since the condition is idiosyncratic, future pregnancy may be entered into with no greater than average risk
d. Fifty percent of patients will completely recover

493. A 78-year-old female presents to your office for follow-up. She has a history of paroxysmal atrial fibrillation and takes warfarin and digoxin for this problem. Her complaints today are a recent 5-lb weight loss, daily fatigue, and loss of interest in her usual activities. She states she doesn't feel like getting up in the morning. Her spouse adds that she has started taking some alternative therapies from the health food store in an attempt to boost her energy level. On exam, the patient is less animated than usual, and her pulse is irregular at 120/min. She has clear lungs and 1+ edema of the lower extremities. You examine the bag of pills the spouse has brought from the medicine cabinet at home. Which medication is most likely contributing to the patient's problem with rapid heart rate?

a. Ginkgo biloba
b. Multivitamin with minerals
c. St. John's wort
d. Soy estrogen
e. Ginseng

494. A 40-year-old female presents to your office regarding a breast lump she found on self-exam 2 weeks ago. The patient does not regularly examine her breasts. Her last clinical breast exam was 2 years ago, and mammogram 9 months ago was normal with recommendation for follow-up mammogram in 1 year. She has no family members with breast cancer. Her father had colon cancer diagnosed 10 years ago. She takes no medications regularly. On examination, she has a well-localized nontender nodule with irregular borders of approximately 1.5 cm in the left breast at 2:00. Repeat diagnostic breast imaging reveals a negative mammogram and solid area at 2:00 in the left breast by ultrasound. Which of the following is the most appropriate next step?

a. Reassure your patient and follow up in 6 months
b. Refer the patient for surgical biopsy
c. Tell the patient to discontinue caffeine and wear a supportive bra
d. Schedule a CT scan of the thorax
e. Start the patient on NSAIDs and vitamin E

495. A 57-year-old white female with a significant past medical history of breast cancer stage 2, ER+, PR+, presents to the emergency room complaining of the sudden onset of chest pain and shortness of breath 2 h ago. The pain is sharp and stabbing in the left posterior lung area. The pain does not increase on exertion but increases with deep breathing. The patient denies any history of cardiovascular or pulmonary disease. Her only medication is tamoxifen for 2 years and OTC vitamins. Pulse is 110, RR 26, BP 150/94; lungs are clear bilaterally; cardiovascular exam shows regular rate and rhythm with a fixed split on S_2. ECG shows S wave in lead I, Q wave in lead III, and inverted T in lead III.

Pulse oximetry is 90% on room air. Chest x-ray is unremarkable. What is most likely to have contributed to this patient's current respiratory distress?

a. Myocardial infarction
b. Breast cancer metastasis
c. Tamoxifen use
d. Anxiety attack
e. Pneumonia

496. A 48-year-old woman presents for her annual exam. She is otherwise healthy. Her main complaint is frequent sweating episodes. These have been intermittent for the past 6 to 9 months. They have gradually worsened. She has three to four flushing/sweating episodes during the day and two to three at night. She occasionally feels her heart race and this lasts about a second, but when she checks her pulse it is normal. She reports feeling more tired and has difficulty with sleep due to sweating. She denies major life stressors. She also denies weight loss, weight gain, or change in bowel habits. Her last menstrual cycle was 12 months ago. She states her quality of life has been affected. You find no abnormalities on physical exam.

Which of the following treatments is the most appropriate choice to alleviate this woman's symptoms?

a. Levothyroxine
b. Estrogen
c. Estrogen plus progesterone
d. Fluoxetine

497. A 67 year old female presents to the emergency room with chest pain that is typical of angina. She is diagnosed with a non–Q wave myocardial infarction. Compared to a similar male patient, which of the following is more likely to occur during this hospital stay in this female patient?

a. Death
b. Need for percutaneous transluminal coronary angioplasty
c. Hypertension
d. Depression

498. A 60-year-old woman presents with complaints of pain during intercourse. She describes the pain as sharp and constant during the sexual activity, and there is a lack of lubrication. Her sex drive has decreased and her husband is upset about this. She underwent surgical menopause at age 44 due to uterine fibroids and pelvic pain. She used oral estrogen until age 50, then stopped. She reports she is attracted to her husband and their marriage is going well. She is active in the community and has several close friends whom she sees regularly. On physical exam you note significant genital and vaginal atrophy. Which of the following is the best treatment option for this patient?

a. Commercial lubricant (K-Y lubricating jelly)
b. Oral estrogen
c. Vaginal estrogen preparation
d. Antidepressant

499. A 32-year-old female G3P3 presents to your office 8 weeks postpartum. She complains of fatigue and neck fullness. Exam reveals a diffusely enlarged thyroid gland, nontender, no focal nodularity. Neuro exam shows a fine tremor. Laboratory evaluation reveals a TSH < 0.01 (normal 0.4 to 4.0) and an elevated total T_4 of 14. A thyroid uptake scan is ordered. You expect to see which of the following?

a. Increased uptake in the thyroid gland
b. Decreased uptake in the thyroid gland
c. Multiple hot nodules
d. Not enough information to determine

500. A 58-year-old female presents to your office for an acute visit pertaining to a sinus infection. She states she takes no medications except a "baby aspirin." When you inquire why she is taking the 81-mg aspirin, she says "to prevent heart attacks." Her history is negative for hypertension, hyperlipidemia, smoking, diabetes, obesity, or family history of cardiovascular disease. What would you advise this patient about the use of aspirin for heart attack prevention?

a. She should take a full-dose aspirin for better cardiovascular protection
b. She does not need to take aspirin for cardiovascular protection
c. She should take a full-dose aspirin every other day
d. She should take an aspirin only if she experiences chest pain

Women's Health

Answers

478. The answer is a. *(Kasper, pp 1056–1057.)* Human papillomavirus (especially subtypes 16, 18, 33, and 45) has an established relationship to abnormal Pap smears and cervical dysplasia. Neither HIV, chlamydia, herpesvirus, or Group B strep infections are directly associated with cervical dysplasia.

479. The answer is a. *(Kasper, pp 27, 2208.)* The current recommendation for workup of abnormal cervical cytology includes repeat Pap smear at 3 to 4 months, HPV DNA typing, or colposcopy, depending on the patient and her history. A Pap smear every 3 years is acceptable for low-risk patients with three negative annual consecutive Pap smears. There is no recommendation for early repeat Pap smear if a patient has a new sexual partner. Sexually active women should have annual cervical screening, with the exception of low-risk patients, who can discuss changing the screening interval with their physician.

480. The answer is b. *(Kasper, pp 2271–2272.)* The World Health Organization and the National Osteoporosis Foundation agree that all postmenopausal patients who are estrogen-deficient with at least one additional risk factor should have a central bone densitometry. A nuclear medicine scan has no role in the diagnosis of osteoporosis. Certainly this patient with estrogen deficiency, low calcium intake, family history, and previous tobacco use has a high pretest probability of osteoporosis; therefore a peripheral bone densitometry, which is used for screening only, would not be a diagnostic test of choice. In addition, due to the above explanation, testing is justified.

481. The answer is b. *(Kasper, pp 2270, 2274–2277.)* Postmenopausal women not on estrogen replacement should achieve a daily intake of calcium at 1200 mg of elemental calcium. The average woman in the United States receives 600 to 700 mg from diet alone. The current recommendation is that women consume 1200 mg oral calcium supplement in two or three divided doses. Although fluoride is an osteoclast inhibitor, early studies revealed an increased fracture rate with fluoride supplementation for prevention or treatment of osteoporosis. Fluoride does not have a proven role in the prevention or treatment of osteoporosis. The current exercise regimen recommended is weight-bearing activities such as walking, dancing, tennis, or jogging three to five times per week. This patient is not performing adequate weight-bearing exercise. There is no indication at this time that the patient should restart hormone replacement therapy. If this patient is diagnosed with osteoporosis, treatment options include the bisphosphonates, calcitonin, and selective estrogen modulators (SERMs). Hormone replacement therapy is not FDA-approved solely for the prevention or treatment of osteoporosis.

482. The answer is e. *(Kasper, pp 2269–2271.)* A positive family history of osteoporosis is a risk factor for the development of osteoporosis. There is a definite relationship between prolonged hyperthyroidism or oversupplementation of hypothyroid patients, but hypothyroidism per se is not associated with the development of osteoporosis. A body weight under 70 kg, not obesity, is associated with osteoporosis. Hormone replacement therapy has been proven to increase bone mineral density and prevent osteoporotic fractures and is therefore not a risk factor in the development of osteoporosis. Vitamin C supplementation at normal or excess amounts has not been linked to the development of osteoporosis.

483. The answer is a. *(Kasper, p 29.)* This patient has exercise-induced symptoms. Women may present with atypical symptoms relating to coronary artery disease. This patient has hyperlipidemia that is untreated and may have type 2 diabetes mellitus with a random glucose of 200 mg/dL. These risk factors coupled with her symptoms make coronary artery disease the most likely choice. This patient's history and physical are negative for signs and symptoms relating to pneumonia. Diuretics do not contribute to dyspnea. The history is not suggestive of anxiety or panic disorder.

484. The answer is d. *(Kasper, pp 29, 1326.)* The most appropriate test would be a graded treadmill stress test with thallium imaging. A graded treadmill stress test has a lower sensitivity and specificity in patients with atypical or no chest pain. A graded treadmill stress test has an increased rate of false-positives and false-negatives in women compared to men. Therefore a negative treadmill stress test would not rule out coronary disease. Subsequent thallium imaging improves sensitivity and specificity. In this patient with hypertension, glucose intolerance, and obesity, the most appropriate first-line evaluation would include ruling out coronary artery disease; therefore pulmonary function testing would not be useful.

485. The answer is b. *(Kasper, p 422.)* Calculated BMI = weight $(kg)/height (m)^2$.

486. The answer is e. *(Kasper, p 422.)* Data from the Metropolitan Life Tables indicate that BMIs for the midpoint of all heights and frames among both men and women range from 19 to 26 kg/m^2. Even at similar BMIs, women have more body fat than men. A BMI of less than 18.5 can precipitate complications from anorexia. The desired BMI range is 18.5 to 24.9.

487. The answer is d. *(Gabbe, pp 1155–1156.)* The patient's clinical presentation is most consistent with postpartum thyroiditis, a form of autoimmune-induced thyrotoxicosis that occurs 3 to 6 months after delivery. The hyperthyroid state usually lasts for 1 to 3 months and is generally followed by a hypothyroid state of limited duration. The patient's thyroid gland would not be enlarged if she were taking exogenous thyroid medications. Subacute thyroiditis almost always presents with a tender, enlarged thyroid gland. The patient's thyroid gland is described as homogeneous, not nodular, which would be inconsistent with toxic multinodular goiter. Struma ovarii is unlikely because of the enlargement of the thyroid gland. Struma ovarii is the name given to the approximately 3% of ovarian dermoid tumors or teratomas that contain thyroid tissue. This tissue may autonomously secrete thyroid hormone. Graves' disease is another possibility. These two abnormal thyroid states could be distinguished with thyroid uptake scan.

488. The answer is b. *(Abelloff, p 2373.)* Recent data from the Women's Health Initiative randomized trial of estrogen and progesterone in healthy postmenopausal women found a 26% increase in the risk of breast cancer over a mean follow-up of 5.2 years. This trial confirmed the benefit of HRT in prevention of osteoporotic fractures, but did not show a benefit in prevention of coronary heart disease. Routine use of postmenopausal HRT for prevention of coronary heart disease is no longer recommended for all women, irrespective of breast cancer risk. Short-term use of post-menopausal HRT (<5 years) for relief of postmenopausal symptoms remains a reasonable option for some women.

489. The answer is e. (*Legato, pp 131, 134.*) This patient's headache pattern is typical of menstrual migraines, occurring within several days of menses. She denies fatigue or stress contributing to headache; therefore tension headache is not likely. She has no aura associated with the headache; therefore classic migraine (migraine with aura) is not correct. Cluster headaches tend to occur in brief, sharp bursts and are more common in men than women. Migraine is precipitated by menstruation in 24 to 68% of women. Although this patient's history points to menstrual migraine, before initiating treatment a headache diary should be recorded for 2 to 3 months to ensure that the migraines occur exclusively or primarily within 3 days of the onset of menses.

490. The answer is a. (*Marx, pp 2408–2409.*) It is important to recognize the increased risk of domestic abuse during pregnancy. In addition, abused pregnant women can have vague physical symptoms, including headache, fatigue, insomnia, choking sensations, gastrointestinal complaints, and pelvic pain. However, jumping to the conclusion that the patient's spouse caused her apparent injuries is not warranted. Often, a patient simply needs the opportunity to express her concerns if she is in an abusive situation.

491. The answer is b. (*Gabbe, p 1667.*) Empiric treatment of simple UTI in pregnancy should consider the following: coverage of probable organisms (usually *Escherichia coli*), possibility of complicating factors such as pyelonephritis or nephrolithiasis, stage of pregnancy, and relative contraindication to the antibiotic. The antibiotics listed all would cover suspected organisms in simple UTI of pregnancy. However, all but one of the antibiotics is contraindicated in pregnancy. Ciprofloxacin is pregnancy category D because of concern about cartilage formation in animal studies. Trimethoprim-sulfa is not the best choice in later stages of pregnancy because trimethoprim is a folate antagonist and is teratogenic in rats, and sulfa drugs have increased risk of kernicterus in premature neonates. Tetracycline is avoided because of possibility of discoloration of teeth and hypoplasia of tooth enamel and long bone growth in the neonate. Also, the mother is at increased risk for acute fatty necrosis of the liver. Gentamicin is not indicated because of concern for possible ototoxicity in the neonate.

492. The answer is d. (*Kasper, pp 1409–1410.*) By definition, peripartum cardiomyopathy is cardiac dilatation and CHF of unexplained cause occurring during the last trimester of pregnancy or within 6 months of delivery. Half of patients will completely recover normal cardiac size and function. However, further pregnancies frequently produce increasing myocardial damage and increased mortality, and patients should be counseled to avoid future pregnancies. Treatment is the same as for other types of dilated cardiomyopathies and includes salt restriction, angiotensin-converting enzyme inhibitors, diuretics, and digitalis and/or beta-blockers for symptomatic treatment. Other treatment modalities may include anticoagulation to prevent systemic embolization and an implantable cardioverter-defibrillator in patients with arrhythmias.

493. The answer is c. (*Gaster, pp 152–156.*) The patient is attempting to self-treat her depressive symptoms with St. John's wort, which has been reported to interact with certain prescription medications, including digoxin. St. John's wort may lower levels of digoxin by 25%. Another interaction that could be important in this case is bleeding, which has been reported in patients taking warfarin and ginkgo biloba.

494. The answer is b. (*Kasper, pp 517–519.*) Palpable breast mass evaluation should determine whether the patient has a true mass or prominent physiologic glandular tissue. The next step is to determine whether the dominant mass represents a cyst, a benign solid mass, or cancer. The physical characteristics of this patient's mass that cause concern include irregular borders, size larger than 1 cm, and location in the upper outer quadrant of the breast. This patient's age (>35) also places her at slightly higher risk. Therefore repeat imaging including ultrasound is warranted. If no cyst is found and mammogram is negative, the patient should be examined by a breast surgeon or a comprehensive breast radiologist and biopsy performed. Six months is too long to reevaluate. In a younger woman (<35), repeat exam after the next menstrual cycle might be warranted (i.e., <1-month reevaluation). To assume breast changes are benign without further investigation is not appropriate. CT scanning does not currently provide useful information in the evaluation of palpable breast mass.

495. The answer is c. *(Kasper, p 1561.)* This patient's history and physical are consistent with a pulmonary embolus. The combination of respiratory distress, hypoxia, tachycardia, clear chest x-ray, and typical ECG changes makes this the most likely choice. There is no evidence on chest x-ray of infiltrate or metastatic disease. An anxiety attack would not cause hypoxia. Tamoxifen is associated with an increased risk of thromboembolic events.

496. The answer is c. *(Stenchever, pp 1227–1228.)* The differential diagnosis for palpitations and sweating is broad but major consideration should be given to hyperthyroidism, panic attacks, cardiac arrythmias, malignancy, and vasomotor instability. This patient denies symptoms of malignancy such as weight loss. She does not have symptoms of clinical depression such as apathy or suicidal thoughts. She reports no change in bowel habits or weight, which would indicate the diagnosis of thyroid disorder. The most likely diagnosis for this patient is vasomotor symptoms due to menopause. The best treatment option for this patient is estrogen plus progesterone. Women who still have a uterus are treated with combination hormone replacement therapy for uterine protection against endometrial carcinoma.

497. The answer is a. *(Legato, p 224.)* Women have higher rates of mortality in the 30 days post-MI. In the setting of an acute MI, women are also more likely to present with congestive heart failure, hypotension, or cardiogenic shock. In addition, women are more likely to undergo major clinical events during hospitalization, including cardiac rupture, atrial fibrillation, and cerebrovascular accidents. The incidence of depression is higher in women. However, it is not widely accepted that women become more depressed after an acute myocardial infarction.

498. The answer is c. *(Stenchever, pp 1227–1228.)* This patient has dyspareunia, or pain during intercourse. She has been postmenopausal for many years and without hormone (estrogen) replacement. A commercial lubricant would be helpful for vaginal dryness but will not treat the underlying disorder of urogenital atrophy, which is due to hypoestrogenemia. She has no other symptoms of menopause that impair quality of life such as vasomotor symptoms or sleep disturbance. Therefore oral estrogen is not required. She denies depressive symptoms. The best treatment option for this patient is to treat the underlying disorder of urogenital atrophy with topical estrogen applied to the vagina. A commercial lubricant could be used as needed, but would be in addition to the vaginal hormone cream.

499. The answer is b. *(Gabbe, pp 1155–1156.)* Postpartum thyroiditis is an autoimmune destruction of the thyroid gland that causes release of already formed hormone. Therefore, uptake in the damaged gland is low. The thyroid scan for thyroiditis shows low RAI uptake versus Graves' disease, where the uptake is increased. In Graves' disease, auto-antibodies bind to the TSH receptor and stimulate the gland to increase function and hormone output. Therefore, in Graves' disease there is increased uptake on the thyroid scan. *Most* cases of postpartum thyroiditis spontaneously recover after 3 to 6 months; watchful waiting is the best approach to this abnormality.

500. The answer is b. *(N Engl J Med 352:1293–1304, 2005. Circulation 109:672–693, 2004.)* This patient is at low risk for cardiovascular disease. Her only listed major cardiovascular risk factor is age >55. The American Heart Association has published "Evidence-based Medicine in the Prevention of Cardiovascular Disease in Women." This guideline recommends that aspirin prophylaxis be used for women at high risk for CVD. In intermediate-risk women aspirin should be taken if blood pressure is controlled and benefit exceeds gastrointestinal risk. In low-risk individuals, aspirin prophylaxis is not recommended. Since the publication of the AHA guidelines in 2004, a large study, "The Women's Health Study," was published *(NEJM, 2005)*. In this study, consisting of more than 39,000 women, aspirin prophylaxis did not provide a significant decrease in myocardial infarction or death from cardiovascular events, although it did decrease the risk of ischemic stroke.

Bibliography

Abelloff MD, Armitage JO, Niederhuber JE, et al (eds): *Clinical Oncology,* 3/e, Philadelphia, Churchill Livingstone, 2004.

Cochran ST: Anaphylactoid reactions to radiocontrast media. *Curr Allergy Asthma Rep* 5(1):28–31, Jan 2005.

Gabbe SG, Neibyl JR, Simpson JL (eds): *Gabbe: Obstetrics—Normal and Problem Pregnancies,* 4/e, Philadelphia, Churchill Livingstone, Inc., 2002.

Gantz NM, Brown RB, Berk SL et al (eds): *Manual of Clinical Problems in Infectious Disease,* 5/e, Philadelphia, Lippincott Williams and Wilkins, 2005.

Gaster B, Holroyd J: St. John's wort for depression. *Arch Int Med* 160:152–156, 2000.

JNC 7 Express. The Seventh Report of the Joint National Committee on Prevention, Detection, Evaluation, and Treatment of High Blood Pressure. National Institutes of Health, National Heart, Lung, and Blood Institute, NIH Publication 03-5233, December 2003. [Also found in *JAMA* 289:2560–2572, 2003.] (www.nhlbi.nih.gov/guidelines/hypertension/express.pdf)

Kane RL, Ouslander JG, Abrass IB: *Essentials of Clinical Geriatrics,* 5/e, New York, McGraw-Hill, 2004.

Kasper DL, Braunwald E, Fauci AS, Hauser SL, et al (eds): *Harrison's Principles of Internal Medicine,* 16/e, New York, McGraw-Hill, 2005.

Legato MJ, *Principles of Gender-Specific Medicine,* 1/e, London UK, Elsevier Press, 2004.

Mandell GL, Bennett JE, Dolin, R (eds): *Principles and Practice of Infectious Diseases,* 5/e, New York, Churchill Livingstone, 2000.

Marx JA, Hockberger RS, Walls RM (eds): *Rosen's Emergency Medicine: Concepts and Clinical Practice,* 5/e, St. Louis MI, Mosby Inc., 2002.

Mosca L et al: Evidence-based guidelines for cardiovascular disease prevention in women. *Circulation* 109:672, 2004.

Ridker PM et al: A randomized trial of low-dose aspirin in the primary prevention of cardiovascular disease in women. *N Engl J Med* 352:1293, 2005.

Sampson HA: Food-induced anaphylaxis. *Novartis Found Symp* 257:161–71; discussion 171–176, 207–210, 276–285, 2004.

Stenchever MA, Droegemueller W, Herbst AL, Mishell DR (eds): *Clinical Oncology*, 3/e, Philadelphia, Churchill Livingstone, 2004.

Stein JH: *Internal Medicine*, 5/e. Boston, Little, Brown & Company, 1998.

Stobo JD, Hellman DB, Ladenson PW et al (eds): *The Principles and Practice of Medicine*, 23/e, Stamford, CT. Appleton & Lange, 1996.

Third Report of the National Cholesterol Education Program (NCEP) Expert Panel on Detection, Evaluation, and Treatment of High Blood Cholesterol in Adults (Adult Treatment Panel III) Executive Summary, National Heart, Lung, and Blood Institute, National Institutes of Health, NIH Publication 01-3670, May 2001. [Also found in *JAMA* 285:2486–2497, 2001.] (www.nhlbi.gov/guidelines/cholesterol/atp3xsum.pdf)

Victor M, Ropper AH: *Adams and Victor's Principles of Neurology*, 7/e, New York, McGraw-Hill, 2001.

Wolff K, Johnson RA, Suurmond D: *Fitzpatrick's Color Atlas & Synopsis of Clinical Dermatology*, 5/e, New York, McGraw-Hill, 2005.

Index

A

Acetaminophen, 305, 311
Achalasia, 157, 169
Acidosis
    metabolic, 178–179, 180, 188–189, 190
    renal tubular, 179, 189
    respiratory, 54, 67, 71, 80
Acne, 251, 263
Acromegaly, 129, 143
Actinomyces israelii, 11, 25
Actinomycosis, cervicofacial, 11, 25
Addison's disease, 126–127, 141–142
Adrenal gland tumor, 130, 143
Adrenal insufficiency, 126–127, 141–142
Agranulocytosis, 207, 223
AIDS (acquired immunodeficiency syndrome), 13–14, 26
Aldosterone, 123, 138
Alkalosis
    metabolic, 180, 189–190
    respiratory, 67, 80, 180, 182, 190, 191
Allergic reactions
    food allergies, 297, 302
    insect stings, 297, 303
    latex, 296, 301
    radiocontrast agents, 296, 301

Allergic reactions (*Cont.*):
    treatment of, 279, 290, 296, 301
    (*See also* Anaphylaxis)
Alzheimer's disease, 236, 248, 305, 311
Amantadine, 12, 21, 25, 315
Amaurosis fugax, 239, 250
Amyotrophic lateral sclerosis, 229, 242–243
Anaerobic infection, 52, 70
Anaphylaxis
    immunoglobulin deficiencies, 296, 301
    treatment of, 296, 301
    (*See also* Allergic reactions)
Anemia
    of chronic disease, 195, 211–212, 225
    diagnosis of, 308, 313–314
    hemolytic, 196, 206, 212, 222
    iron-deficiency, 209, 225
    megaloblastic, 206, 222
    microcytic, 195, 211
    of renal disease, 209, 225
    sideroblastic, 209, 212, 225
Angina, 83, 84, 104, 105
Angiotensin-converting enzyme inhibitors, 182, 191
Ankylosing spondylitis, 32, 36, 38, 43, 48, 50–51
Anorexia nervosa, 320, 330

Anthrax, 261, 268
Antiarrhythmia management, 101, 116
Antibiotic therapy
  adverse effects, 15, 27
  methicillin-resistant *Staphylococcus aureus* (MRSA), 8, 21
  mycoplasma infections, 3, 18
  pelvic inflammatory disease, 5, 19
  Pneumocystis carinii, 10, 23
  prophylactic treatment, 9, 23
  sexually transmitted diseases, 2, 5, 14–15, 17–18, 19, 27
Antimalarial drugs, 206, 222
Antiviral agents, 12, 25
Aortic aneurysm, abdominal, 89, 109
Aortic dissection, 91, 110
Aortic regurgitation, 100, 115
Aortic stenosis, 86, 107
Aortoenteric fistula, 160, 161, 172
Arrhenoblastoma, 132, 144–145
Arsenic poisoning, 278, 289
Arthritis
  osteoarthritis, 31, 42–43, 305, 311
  psoriatic, 34, 45
  rheumatoid, 29, 35, 40, 47–48
  septic, 30–31, 41–42
Asbestosis, 69, 82
Aspergillus flavus, 16, 28
Aspergillus fumigatus, 12, 13, 25
Aspirin prophylaxis, 327, 334
Asthma, 56, 58, 72, 75
Atelectasis, 61, 77
Atrial fibrillation, 88, 108–109
Atrial flutter, 98, 113–114
Autonomy, principle of, 278, 279, 289, 290

B
Back pain, 31, 42
Barrett's esophagus, 166

Basilar artery, 239, 250
Behçet syndrome, 38, 50
Berylliosis, 68, 81
Beta blockers, 272, 285
Bladder cancer, 201, 217–218
Blastomycosis dermatitidis, 12, 25
Blood gases, 67, 80
Blood pressure recommendations, 271, 284
Body mass index (BMI), 320, 330
Bone density testing, 318, 328
Bone marrow production problem, 199, 215–216
Bradycardia, sinus, 101, 116
Brain abscess, 236–237, 249
Brainstem lesions, 233, 245
Breast cancer, 133, 145, 208–209, 221, 224–225, 275–276, 288
Breast masses, 205, 221, 324, 332–333
Bronchiectasis, 61, 77–78
Bronchitis, 59, 75
Brown recluse spider bites, 278, 290

C
CAGE questionnaire, 276, 288
Calcium pyrophosphate dihydrate deposition disease (CPPDD), 44, 45–46
Calcium supplements, 318, 328–329
Campylobacter jejuni, 287
Cancers
  basal cell carcinoma, 260, 267
  bladder, 201, 217–218
  breast, 133, 145, 208–209, 221, 224–225, 275–276, 288
  lung, 68, 81, 196, 199, 213, 215
  mucin-producing, 225
  oat cell carcinomas, 210, 226
  ovarian, 200, 216

Cancers (Cont.):
  screening tests, 275–276, 287–288
  skin, 255, 257, 265
  small cell carcinomas, 68, 81, 255,
    265
  squamous, 225–226
  testicular, 208–209, 224
Candida albicans, 16, 27–28
Carbon monoxide poisoning, 62, 78
Cardiac risks, surgery and, 276, 288
Cardiac tamponade, 96, 113
Cardiomyopathy
  hypertrophic, 100, 115–116
  peripartum, 85, 107, 323, 332
Cardiovascular disease, 327, 334
Carotid disease, 239, 250
Carotid sinus hypersensitivity, 227,
  240
Carpal tunnel syndrome, 37, 50
Cerebellar lesions, 246
Cerebral arteries, 239, 250
Cerebrovascular disease, 239, 250
Chemotherapy agents, 208–209,
  224–225
Chickenpox, 9, 23
Chlamydia trachomatis, 11, 14, 19, 24,
  27
Cholangitis, sclerosing, 159, 171
Cholecystitis, 158, 170
Cholesterol, 272, 273, 284, 285–286
Cholesterol embolization, 39, 51
Cigarette smoking
  bladder cancer, 201, 217–218
  carcinomas, 199, 215
  cessation program, 59, 75
Clostridium difficile, 156, 168–169
Cluster headaches, 227, 237, 238, 240,
  246, 249
Cocaine use, 277, 289
Coccidioides immitis, 16, 28

Colitis, 161, 172–173
Colon polyps, 151, 164
Coma
  causes of, 234, 247
  hyperosmolar, 119, 136
  myxedema, 127, 142
Complement deficiencies, 298, 299,
  303, 304
Condyloma acuminatum, 12, 25
Coronary artery disease, 312, 319,
  329–330
Coronary artery occlusions, 83, 104
Coronavirus, 6, 20
Cor pulmonale, 97, 113
Coxsackievirus B, 16, 28
Creutzfeldt-Jakob disease, 236, 248
Crohn's disease, 161, 172
Cryoglobulinemia, 184, 193
Cryptosporidium, 13–14, 26
Cushing's disease, 134, 146
Cystic fibrosis, 68, 80–81
Cytomegalovirus, 13–14, 26
Cytomegalovirus retinitis, 12, 13–14,
  25, 26

D
Decay-accelerating factor deficiency,
  298, 303
Dementia, 236, 248, 306, 311–312
Depression, 277, 288–289, 324, 332
Dermatitis, contact, 253, 263–264
Dermatitis, seborrheic, 258, 267
Dermatomyositis, 245
Desmopressin, 199, 214–215
Diabetes insipidus, 133, 145
Diabetes mellitus
  exercise and, 124, 139
  hypertension and, 271, 284
  management of, 120, 124, 137, 139
  myocardial infarction, 83, 104–105

Diabetes mellitus (*Cont.*):
  pancreatitis, 155, 168
  Somogyi phenomenon, 128, 142
Diabetic ketoacidosis, 67, 80
Diabetic neuropathy, 231, 244
Diarrhea, osmotic, 154, 167
Disease-modifying antirheumatic
  drugs, 40, 47–48
Disseminated intravascular
  coagulation, 207, 222–223
Diuretics, 271, 282, 284, 292, 308,
  314
Diverticulitis, 158, 159, 170–171
Domestic abuse, 323, 331
Duodenal ulcers, 150, 154, 163, 167
Dyspareunia, 326, 333–334

E
Eczema, 269
Elderly patients (*see* Geriatric
  patients)
Empty sella syndrome, 134, 146–147
Empyema, 63, 79
Encephalopathy
  hepatic, 152, 165
  hypertensive, 91, 110–111
Endocarditis
  bacterial, 11, 24–25
  prophylactic treatment, 99, 114
Epiglottitis, 1, 17
Epilepsy, 249–250
Epinephrine, 279, 290
Epstein-Barr virus, 13, 26
Erysipelas, 10, 24
Erythema infectiosum, 13, 25–26
Erythema multiforme, 256, 265
Erythema nodosum, 254, 264
Escherichia coli, 8, 22, 287
Esophageal carcinomas, 153, 165

Exercise recommendations
  diabetic patients, 124, 139
  geriatric patients, 307, 312
  walking, 307, 312
Extracellular fluid, 183, 192

F
Factitious diseases, 23, 133, 146
Fat embolism, 54, 70
Fatty liver, 158, 169–170
Felty's syndrome, 35, 47
Fever of unknown origin (FUO), 9,
  22–23
Fibromyalgia, 34, 37, 46, 49
Fifth disease, 13, 25–26
Focal lesions, 246
Food allergies, 297, 302
Food poisoning, 162, 173
Fungal agents, 12–13, 25

G
Gallstones, 158, 170
Ganciclovir, 12, 25
Gastric ulcers, 160, 172
Gastrinoma, 133, 145, 167
Gastroesophageal reflux disease, 153,
  165–166
Gastropathy, NSAID, 36, 48
Geriatric patients
  exercise recommendations, 307, 312
  immunization recommendations,
    308, 314
  medication recommendations, 307,
    313
  myocardial infarction, 83, 104–105
  physiologic parameters, 308,
    313–314
  restraint use, 306, 312
  tuberculosis and, 283, 292–293

Giant cell arteritis (*see* Temporal arteritis)
Giardia lamblia (giardiasis), 163, 173, 274, 286–287
Glomerular diseases, 183–184, 192–193
Glomerulonephritis, membranoproliferative, 183–184, 193
Glomerulosclerosis, focal, 183–184, 192
Glucose-6–phosphate dehydrogenase deficiency, 160, 171, 222
Gonadotropin-releasing hormone (GnRH), 203, 219
Goodpasture syndrome, 56, 71–72
Gout, 30, 41, 279, 290
Gram stain, 8, 21–22
Granulocytopenia, 35, 47
Grave's disease, 122, 135, 137–138, 147, 207, 223, 334
Guillain-Barré syndrome, 230–231, 243–244

H

Haemophilus influenzae, 17, 304
Hantavirus pulmonary syndrome, 16, 28
Hearing loss, 307, 313
Heart block
    AV block, 90, 98, 109, 113–114
    complete block, 93, 111–112
Heart disease
    endocarditis prophylaxis, 99, 114
    risk factors, 281, 291
    treatment of, 102–103, 117–118
Heart failure, congestive
    chest x-ray, 65, 66, 79
    Framingham criteria, 84, 106

Heart failure, congestive (*Cont.*):
    pleural effusions, 56, 63, 71, 78
    treatment of, 85, 106, 291–292
Heart murmurs and sounds
    paradoxical splitting of S_2, 99, 114
    ventricular septal defect, 87, 108
Helicobacter pylori infection, 150, 163–164
Hematocrit, 308, 313–314
Hematuria, 201, 217–218
Hemianopsia, 129, 143
Hemiplegia, 233, 245
Hemochromatosis, 33, 44, 132, 143–144, 155, 167, 204, 220
Hemoptysis, 69, 81–82
Heparin, 203, 219–220
Hepatic encephalopathy, 152, 165
Hepatitis, viral, 160, 171
Hepatitis B vaccines, 154, 166
Hepatitis C, 156, 169
Hepatocellular carcinoma, 200, 204, 216, 220
Herpes genitalis, 15, 27
Herpes simplex virus, 16, 28
Herpesvirus, human, 262, 270
Herpes zoster, 5, 19
Hip fractures, 35, 46–47
HIV (human immunodeficiency virus)
    manifestations of, 13–14, 26–27
    tuberculosis and, 283, 292–293
    vaccinations and, 275, 287
Hives (*see* Urticaria)
Hodgkin's disease, 68, 81, 202, 218
Hormone replacement therapy (HRT), 322, 325–326, 330–331, 333–334
Human papillomavirus, 317, 328
Huntington's disease, 235, 248
Hyperbilirubinemia, 150, 160, 164, 171

Hypercalcemia, 210, 225–226
Hypercapnia, 67, 80
Hyperglycemia, 119–120, 136–137
Hyperglycemic hyperosmolar
    nonketotic state, 120, 136–137
Hyperkalemia, 103, 117, 181, 191
Hypernatremia, 115
Hyperparathyroidism, 125, 140
Hypertension
    blood pressure recommendations,
        271, 284
    chest x-ray, 66, 67, 80
    diastolic, 123, 138
    malignant, 91, 110–111
    portal, 152, 164–165
    pulmonary hypertension, 60, 76–77,
        97, 113
    refractory, 96, 112
    strokes and, 232, 244
    treatment of, 102–103, 116–117,
        182, 191, 271, 281–282, 284,
        291–292, 308, 314
Hypertensive crisis, 128, 142–143
Hyperthyroidism, 122, 135, 137–138,
    147
Hyperuricemia, 290
Hypoaldosteronism, hyporeninemic,
    181, 190–191
Hypocalcemia, 103, 117
Hypoglycemia, 133, 146, 234, 247
Hypokalemia, 103, 117
Hypomagnesemia, 182, 191
Hyponatremia, 99, 115, 183, 192,
    210, 226
Hypoparathyroidism, 103, 117
Hypophosphatemia, 182, 191
Hypotension, 307, 312–313
Hypothermia, 115
Hypothyroidism, 123, 126, 128,
    138–139, 141, 142

Hypoventilation, 67, 80
Hypoxia, 67, 80

I

Idioventricular rhythm, 101, 116
Immunizations
    for adults, 275, 287
    for geriatric patients, 308, 309,
        314–315
    for HIV-infected patients, 275, 287
Immunodeficiency syndrome, 295,
    300
Immunoglobulin deficiencies, 296,
    301
Immunologic deficiencies, 298–299,
    303–304
Impotence, 124, 139–140
Inappropriate ADH secretion, 129,
    143, 181, 190, 210, 226
Incontinence, 310, 315
Infectious mononucleosis, 4, 13, 18,
    26
Influenza A, 7, 12, 21, 25
Influenza vaccine, 309, 314–315
Insect stings, 297, 303
Interferon α, 12, 25
Interferon β, 228, 241
Intestinal obstructions, 158, 159, 171
Iron storage disorders, 132, 143–144,
    155, 167
Irritable bowel syndrome, 155, 168
Isoniazid treatment, 283, 292–293
Isotretinoin, 251, 263

J

Jaundice, 150, 160, 164, 171–172

K

Kaposi's sarcoma, 262, 270
Keratoses, actinic, 262, 269

Keratoses, seborrheic, 309, 314
Kidney stones, 125, 140, 185, 193
Klinefelter syndrome, 131, 143

L

Laryngeal carcinoma, 68, 81
Latex allergies, 296, 301
Laxative abuse, 154, 167
Lead poisoning, 234, 247
Leukemia, 198, 206, 214, 222
Leukoplakia, 204, 220–221
Lewy body dementia, 306, 311–312
Lithium intoxication, 228, 240–241
Liver abscesses, amebic, 5, 18–19
Liver cirrhosis, 152, 159, 164–165,
    171, 200, 204, 216, 220
Liver dysjunction, 150, 164
Living wills, 279, 290
Lumbar disc herniation, 42
Lungs and lung diseases
    cancers and lymphomas, 68, 81,
        196, 199, 210, 213, 215, 226
    lung tumor, 69, 81–82
    oat cell carcinomas, 210, 226
    obstructive lung diseases, 58, 75
    rheumatoid lung disease, 63, 79
Lupus erythematosus, systemic (SLE),
    32, 43, 184, 193
Lyme disease, 6, 20
Lymphadenopathy, 202, 218, 254,
    264, 295, 300
Lymphoma, 63, 79

M

Malabsorption, 153, 166, 168
Marfan's syndrome, 100, 115
Measles (rubeola), 258, 266
Medical nutrition therapy, 120, 137
Medication errors, 280, 291
Melanomas, 208–209, 224, 257, 265

Meningitis, cryptococcal, 236, 248
Menopause, 325–326, 333–334
Mesothelioma, 63, 79
Metabolic syndrome, 281, 291
Methanol intoxication, 178, 188–189
Methicillin-resistant *Staphylococcus
    aureus* (MRSA), 8, 21
Microalbuminuria, 182, 191
Migraine headaches, 233, 245–246,
    322, 331
Minimal change disease, 183–184, 193
Mitral valve insufficiency, 9, 23
Mitral valve prolapse, 98, 114
Mitral valve stenosis, 86, 107–108
MRSA (methicillin-resistant
    Staphylococcus aureus), 8, 21
Mucormycosis, 25
Multiple endocrine neoplasia (MEN)
    type II, 132, 144
Multiple sclerosis, 228, 241
Myasthenia gravis, 15, 27, 230, 243
Mycoplasma pneumoniae, 3, 18, 196, 212
Myelodysplastic syndrome, 206, 222
Myeloma, 196, 212–213
Myeloproliferative syndrome, 205, 221
Myocardial infarction
    painless or silent, 83, 104–105
    post-cardiac injury syndrome, 84,
        105–106
    presentation of, 94–95, 112
    prevention of, 272, 285
    treatment of, 94, 112, 306, 311
    women and, 326, 333
Myocarditis, 16, 28

N

Neisseria gonorrhoeae, 14, 19, 27
Neisseria meningitidis, 13, 26
Nephropathy, membranous, 183–184,
    192–193

Nephrotic syndrome, 180, 190
Neutropenia, 299, 304
Nonsteroidal anti-inflammatory drugs,
　36, 48, 160, 172

O
Optic neuritis, 228, 241
Osteoarthritis, 31, 42–43, 305, 311
Osteoarthropathy, hypertrophic, 53, 70
Osteoporosis, 125, 140, 318, 328–329
Otitis, malignant external, 1, 17
Ovaries
　arrhenoblastoma, 132, 144–145
　cancer, 200, 216

P
Paget's disease, 124, 126, 134,
　140–141, 146
Pancreatic carcinoma, 160, 171, 225
Pancreatitis, 149, 155, 163, 168, 273,
　286
Pancytopenia, 199, 215–216
Panic disorder, 274, 286
Pap smears, 317, 328
Paracentesis, 152, 164–165
Paraneoplastic syndromes, 210,
　225–226
Parathormone-related peptide,
　225–226
Parathyroid hormone, 182, 191
Parkinson's disease, 234, 235,
　246–247, 248
Parvovirus B19, 13, 25–26
Pelvic inflammatory disease, 5, 19
Peptic ulcer disease, 133, 145, 149,
　150, 163–164
Pericarditis, 96, 112–113, 176, 187,
　274, 286
Phenytoin, 256, 265

Pheochromocytoma, 128, 142–143,
　144
Pituitary tumor, 130, 143
Pityriasis rosea, 258, 266
Plasma osmolality, 178, 188–189
Pleural effusions, 53, 56, 63, 70, 71,
　78–79
Pneumococcal vaccine, 308, 314
Pneumocystis jiroveci (formerly *carinii*),
　10, 13–14, 23–24, 26
Pneumonia
　pneumococcal, 57, 72–73
　Staphylococcus aureus, 64, 66, 79
　Streptococcus pneumoniae, 8, 11,
　　21–22, 25, 57, 72–73
Pneumonitis, hypersensitivity, 297,
　302
Pneumothorax, 59, 75
Poliovirus vaccines, 275, 287
Polyarteritis, microscopic, 39, 51
Polyarteritis nodosa, 38, 39, 50, 51,
　184, 193
Polycythemia vera, 205, 221
Polymyalgia rheumatica, 38, 45, 50
Polymyositis, 233, 244–245
Polysomnography, 60, 77
Post-cardiac injury syndrome, 84,
　105–106
Postmenopausal women, 318,
　328–329
Pregnancy, 323, 331–332
Presbycusis, 307, 313
Prolactinomas, 134, 146
Propylthiouracil, 207, 223
Prostatic carcinoma, 202–203,
　218–219
Providencia stuartii, 11, 25
Pseudogout, 33, 34, 44, 45–46
Pseudomonas aeruginosa, 1, 17, 264

Psoriasis, 252, 263
Psoriatic arthritis, 34, 45
Pulmonary capillary wedge pressure,
    59, 76
Pulmonary embolus, 57–58, 67,
    73–75, 80, 325, 333
Pulmonary function testing, 56, 71–72
Pulsus paradoxus, 56, 72, 96, 113
Purpura, thrombotic
    thrombocytopenic, 197, 213–214

R
Radiocontrast agent sensitivity, 296,
    301
Reiter's syndrome, 33, 44
Renal carcinoma, 200, 216
Renal disease, anemia of, 209, 225
Renal failure
    atheroembolic, 177, 187
    drug-induced, 177, 187–188
    pericarditis, 176, 187
    rhabdomyolysis-induced, 175–176,
        186–187
Renal insufficiency, 103, 117
Renin, 123, 138
Respiratory distress syndrome, adult,
    28, 59, 75–76
Respiratory syncytial virus infection,
    12, 25
Restless leg syndrome, 229, 242
Restraint use, 306, 312
Retinitis, cytomegalovirus, 12, 13–14,
    25, 26
Rheumatic fever, 92, 111
Rheumatoid arthritis, 29, 35, 40,
    47–48
Rheumatoid lung disease, 63, 79
Rhinitis, allergic, 295, 300
Ribavirin, 12, 25

Rocky Mountain spotted fever, 10, 24,
    252, 263
Rosacea, 259, 267
Rubeola (measles), 258, 266

S
Salmonella, 13–14, 26, 173, 287
Sarcoidosis, 55, 71, 254, 264
Sarcomas, soft tissue, 208, 223–224
SARS (severe acute respiratory
    syndrome), 6, 20
Schirmer test, 30, 41
Sciatica, 42
Scleroderma, 32, 43–44
Scrotal mass, 201, 217
Scurvy, 254, 264–265
Seizures
    drug-induced, 15, 27
    types of, 238, 249–250
Sepsis, 59, 75–76, 299, 304
Serum osmolarity, 119, 136
Severe acute respiratory syndrome
    (SARS), 6, 20
Sexually transmitted diseases, 14–15,
    27
Shigella dysenteriae, 162, 173, 287
Sickle cell disease, 11, 25, 205, 221
Sjögren syndrome, 30, 41
Skin abnormalities, 262, 269, 309, 314
Skin cancers, 255, 257, 265
Sleep apnea syndrome, 60–61, 77
Smallpox, 261, 268
Smallpox vaccine, 261, 268–269
Somogyi phenomenon, 128, 142
Spider bites, 278, 290
Spinal cord compression, 201,
    216–217
Spleen, 299, 304
Splenomegaly, 205, 221

Spondyloarthropathies, 32, 43
Sputum Gram stain and culture, 8,
    21–22
Staphylococcus aureus
    food poisoning, 162, 173
    methicillin-resistant *Staphylococcus
        aureus* (MRSA), 8, 21
    pneumonia, 64, 66, 79
    septic arthritis, 31, 42
    toxic shock syndrome, 13, 26
Steatohepatitis, nonalcoholic, 170
St. John's wort, 324, 332
Streptococcus pneumoniae, 8, 11, 21–22,
    25, 57, 72–73
Streptococcus pyogenes, 10, 24
Stress tests, 86, 107, 319, 329–330
Strokes, 232, 244, 247
Subarachnoid hemorrhage, 227, 240
Superior vena cava syndrome, 196,
    213
Surgery, cardiac risks and, 276, 288
Syphilis, 2, 15, 17–18, 27
Systemic lupus erythematosus (SLE),
    32, 43, 184, 193

T
Tachycardia, supraventricular, 89, 93,
    109, 111
Takayasu's arteritis, 39, 52
Tamoxifen, 325, 333
Telangiectasia, hereditary hemorrhagic,
    160, 161, 172
Temporal arteritis, 33, 39, 45, 51–52,
    237, 238, 246, 249
Tension headaches, 237–238, 249
Testicular cancer, 208–209, 224
Testicular mass, 201, 217
Tetanus-diphtheria booster,
    275, 287

Thrombocytopenia, 197, 203,
    213–214, 219–220
Thrombophlebitis, 210, 225
Thymomas, 230, 243
Thyroid gland
    medullary carcinoma, 132, 144
    nodules, 123, 132, 139, 144
    surgery, 103, 117, 138
Thyroiditis
    autoimmune, 123, 126, 138–139,
        141
    postpartum, 321, 326, 330, 334
    subacute, 135, 147
Thyroid peroxidase, 123, 126,
    138–139, 141
Thyrotoxicosis, 121, 137
Tinea corporis, 262, 269
Tinea versicolor, 259, 267
Tinel's sign, 50
Toxic shock syndrome, 7, 13, 20–21, 26
Toxoplasma gondii, 13–14, 26–27
Transfusion reactions, 208, 223
Trichomoniasis, 15, 27
Tricuspid regurgitation, 100, 115
Triglycerides, 273, 286
Trousseau syndrome, 210, 225
Tuberculosis
    adrenal glands and, 126, 141
    chest x-ray, 65, 67, 79–80
    presentation of, 69, 81
    treatment of, 283, 292–293
Tubular necrosis, acute, 15, 27
Tumor necrosis factor (TNF) inhibitors,
    34, 36, 45, 48

U
Urinary tract infections, 11, 25, 323,
    331–332
Urticaria, 253, 254, 264, 295, 300

V

Vaccinations (*see* Immunizations)
Vaccinia necrosum, 261, 268–269
Varicella virus, 9, 23
Vasculitis, 184, 193
Venereal Disease Research Laboratory
    (VDRL) test, 2, 17
Ventricular fibrillation, 90, 110
Ventricular premature complexes, 87,
    101, 108, 116
Ventricular septal defect, 87, 108
Viridans streptococci, 11, 24–25
Vitamin B$_{12}$ deficiency, 197, 206, 214,
    222
von Willebrand's disease, 199,
    214–215

W

Warfarin, 58, 74–75, 88, 108–109,
    204, 220, 277, 289
Wegener's granulomatosis, 37, 48–49,
    184, 193
Wenckebach phenomenon, 90, 109
Wilson's disease, 235, 247–248
Wiskott-Aldrich syndrome, 298,
    303–304

X

Xanthoma, 257, 265–266

Z

Zollinger-Ellison syndrome, 154, 167
Zygomycosis, 12, 13, 25

Notes

Notes

Notes

Notes

Notes

Notes

Notes